'In this book, Berg claims that evidence-based practice in psychology distorts psychotherapy. This bold claim is proven valid throughout the book. It shows that there is a need for a reconstruction of the policy-statement. The book is well written and crystal clear in the presentation of philosophical concepts and in the analysis of evidence-based practice in psychology.'

Henrik Eriksen, *Danish Psychological Association*

A Critical Reconstruction of Evidence-based Practice in Psychology

Evidence-based practice in psychology is the dominant regulatory principle in clinical psychology, defining psychological knowledge and its application. This book provides a critical analysis and a reconstruction of the policy statement focusing on epistemology and ethics.

The book shows the ideological and historical background for the development of evidence-based practice in psychology. It covers the main conceptual and empirical arguments leading to this transition including philosophy and evidence-based medicine. The book goes on to show some of the defects of evidence-based practice in psychology: it misconstrues psychological knowledge; reduces the number of ethical resources available to regulate psychological practices; does not fulfil its ambitions of being a tripartite concept; and undertheorises the issue of integration. The closing chapters provide a constructive critique, preserving the valuable aspects of evidence-based practice in psychology while developing it to make it function adequately. In that sense, the book aims to change the way psychological knowledge is understood and used in practice.

This text will be engaging and thought-provoking for anyone using psychological knowledge with patients or clients. It will provide analytic resources to understand psychology better and facilitate the application of psychological knowledge in various settings.

Henrik Berg, PhD, is a full professor in theory of science at the University of Bergen. He has an academic background in philosophy and psychology. He also is a clinical psychologist.

Routledge Focus on Mental Health

Routledge Focus on Mental Health presents short books on current topics, linking in with cutting-edge research and practice.

Titles in the series:

Life Skills and Adolescent Mental Health: Can Kids Be Taught to Master Life?
Ole Jacob Madsen

Gender, Sexuality and Subjectivity: A Lacanian Perspective on Identity, Language and Queer Theory
Duane Rousselle

Lacan, Jouissance and the Social Sciences: The One and the Many
Raul Moncayo

Understanding and Coping with Illness Anxiety
Phil Lane

The Linguistic Turn of the English Renaissance: A Lacanian Perspective
Shirley Zisser

The Concept of the Individual in Psychoanalysis: The Ego, the Self, the Subject, and the Person
Raul Moncayo

A Critical Reconstruction of Evidence-based Practice in Psychology: Evidence and Ethics
Henrik Berg

For a full list of titles in this series, please visit https://www.routledge.com/Routledge-Focus-on-Mental-Health/book-series/RFMH

A Critical Reconstruction of Evidence-based Practice in Psychology

Evidence and Ethics

Henrik Berg

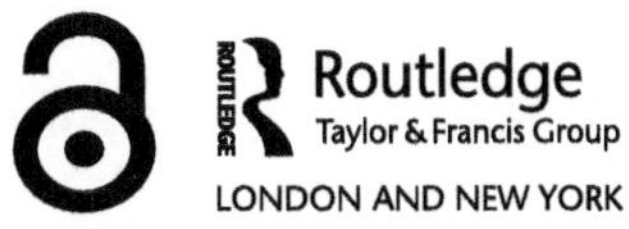

First published 2025
by Routledge
4 Park Square, Milton Park, Abingdon, Oxon OX14 4RN

and by Routledge
605 Third Avenue, New York, NY 10158

Routledge is an imprint of the Taylor & Francis Group, an informa business

British Library Cataloguing-in-Publication Data
A catalogue record for this book is available from the British Library

ISBN: 978-1-032-84297-4 (hbk)
ISBN: 978-1-032-84299-8 (pbk)
ISBN: 978-1-003-51214-1 (ebk)

DOI: 10.4324/9781003512141

Typeset in Times New Roman
by SPi Technologies India Pvt Ltd (Straive)

Contents

1 Introduction

Psychology is a major part of current culture and society. Parents receive professional advice based on attachment theory. Both childcare workers and teachers are taught psychology to contribute towards children's development. Many places, standardised health, safety, and environment routines are established to improve work-life satisfaction and performance. If you suffer from mental distress or illness, you can seek professional help. In addition, the number of self-help books is increasing by the minute and psychotherapy has become a part of popular culture through movies and television shows. In short, psychology matters to how we understand ourselves and others.

But how well do we really understand psychology and its effects? The German philosopher Friedrich Nietzsche (1844–1900) argued that deeply held cultural presuppositions must be uncovered through analysis (Ricoeur, 1970). When something does not merely surround us, but partly defines us, we tend to develop blind spots that prevent understanding (Nietzsche, 2012). Consequently, it is sometimes easier to understand other historical eras or cultures because their perspective differs from ours. Maybe, then, we have taken for granted a way of conceptualising psychology which is problematic on closer scrutiny.

The main theme of this book is problems relating to the policy statement for evidence-based practice in psychology. The policy statement was launched by the American Psychological Association. The American Psychological Association (2006) defines evidence-based practice in psychology as 'integration of the best available research with clinical expertise in the context of patient characteristics, culture, and preferences' (p. 1127). Evidence-based practice in psychology defines the proper use of psychological knowledge. It is arguably the single most important document for psychotherapists. However, the influence is not limited to determining which interventions psychotherapists are using. The policy statement also affects how other professionals, politicians, and lay people think about psychology. As psychology and psychotherapy affects how we think about ourselves, our self-understanding is at stake.

DOI: 10.4324/9781003512141-1

Unsurprisingly, scientific findings are central in evidence-based practice in psychology. Thus, an important task is to characterise psychology. This text is critical by nature. Nonetheless, it maintains that scientific findings should inform psychological practices like psychotherapy. The aim is to let science inform decisions in an optimal manner. That, in turn, requires a good understanding of the nature of science. One of the most basic themes in the philosophy of science is the demarcation of science (Popper, 1963, 2014). The question of demarcation is related to the question of how science should inform practices like psychotherapy. However, to answer such questions, we need knowledge about science and the nature of the practice in question (here psychotherapy).

The introduction of the term 'science' raises some fundamental questions. Is psychology *one* science or does it consist of several (parallel) scientific traditions? If it is comprised by several traditions, do they share the same goal? These are, of course, complex questions requiring detailed analyses. There are several different objects of inquiry that naturally belongs to psychology. It includes everything from nerve cells to cultures. Moreover, psychology is methodically pluralistic. It includes natural and social science as well as humanistic research. Judging by the topics and methods in scientific journals, at least, psychology is a diverse discipline.

Let us start by outlining some basic features of science. Science provides simplified descriptions or theories about the world. Theories provide systematic analyses of one (or several) objects of inquiry. They should be transparent enough for others to obtain an understanding of the premises and inferences in the theories. If science works properly, the theories provide a better understanding of the object of study. However, scientific theories are always simplifications of a complex reality. Consequently, it is crucial that the relation between the model and the complex reality is thematised. This is as important when scientific models are used in practice. Thus, philosophy of science, which analyses the relation between theories and (a complex) reality (Sellars, 1963), is a critical resource to turn scientific knowledge into best possible practice (Feyerabend, 2010).

Psychology and the pursuit of the good

A scientific foundation does not guarantee the ethical goodness of psychological practices. Cynical (scientifically informed) actors may use psychology for manipulation. Market actors may, for example, use knowledge about how to influence children to sell their products at the highest possible price (Moore, 2004). More dramatically, scientific knowledge of pain circuits can inform torture in warfare. The combination of science and technology can manipulate the population in democracies. The fact that psychological theories are scientific makes them (rather well-documented) resources that may be used for better or worse. The theories themselves may have implicit ends, but these are rarely made explicit. As an example, a psychological theory which describes human aggression may have reducing aggression as an implicit goal. However, it does not typically explain why this objective is a good objective (Anderson & Bushman, 2002). Such discussions are not a part of certain conceptions of science and must thus be discussed by means of other kinds of analysis. Normally such analyses belong to ethics, which is central to the understanding of psychology and psychotherapy. Thus, ethics (as will be shown) is central to understand the presuppositions and effects of evidence-based practice in psychology.

Over-generalised science can have detrimental consequences. This problem is particularly relevant in complex sciences, which both psychology and psychotherapy exemplify. Science may pathologise an overextensive proportion of human life. This has its own term – medicalisation. Medicalisation designates whenever our concern with pathology has become overextensive. Medicalisation causes human suffering through causing a disproportionate fear of illness (Maturo, 2012). The term 'medicalisation' illustrates that good intentions (such as reducing humans suffering) may paradoxically cause suffering. The risk of good intentions leading to bad consequences only grow with increased complexity (Hacking, 1999). Incorporating sufficient complexity in our analyses is thus required for science to result in the best possible practical consequences.

Evidence-based practice in psychology primarily intends to regulate practical use of psychological knowledge. In other words, it provides a definition of best psychological practice – first and foremost psychotherapy. Yet, the implications exceed this aim. The policy statement impacts the relationship to adjacent disciplines. Evidence-based practice in psychology also provides authorities with an instrument to design and regulate services. Moreover, it affects knowledge production through providing epistemic standards. One example is what methods are being used in research. Another is what type of projects that receive research funding from funding agencies. In addition, it affects the understanding of the expert and patient roles, which influence practices. Finally, evidence-based practice in psychology guides how we understand psychotherapy. One of the main themes in this book is that evidence-based practice in psychology implies a conceptualisation of psychotherapy which fails to capture its distinctive character.

The chapters of the book

The policy statement for evidence-based practice in psychology was formulated somewhat recently. However, the basis for the policy statement is constituted by various pre-existing epistemic and political ideals. Criticisms of evidence-based practice in psychology should not be confined to the specific content of the policy statement. It should also include its presuppositions. By placing evidence-based practice in psychology in ideological, political, and historical context, some of the problems pertaining to it may become clearer. These topics are covered in Chapter 2.

There is a more internal genesis of evidence-based practice in psychology. In this genesis, the history of medicine is central, resulting in evidence-based medicine. The policy statement for evidence-based practice in psychology is explicitly moulded on evidence-based medicine (evidence-based medicine forms the template for evidence-based practice in psychology). As their histories are intertwined, the history of evidence-based medicine is relevant for understanding evidence-based practice in psychology. This will be recapitulated in Chapter 3.

The development of evidence-based practice in psychology must also be linked to the history of psychology and psychotherapy. Here, the establishing of empirically validated treatments is particularly important. In combination with evidence-based medicine, it constitutes (a significant part of) the historical background for evidence-based practice in psychology. By the same token, evidence-based practice in psychology arose as a critique of empirically validated treatments. Chapter 4 describes this development and how evidence-based practice in psychology is defined.

Psychotherapy aims to reduce human suffering. In other words, there is an intention of doing 'good' at the very core of psychotherapy. Whether psychotherapy is a well-suited instrument to obtain certain goals can be informed by science. However, science is not sufficient to determine whether an end is desirable. To find an answer to this question, we must look outside the traditional boundaries of science and introduce ethics. A fundamental theme throughout the book is the many ways in which evidence-based practice in psychology marginalises the role of ethics in psychotherapy. The consequence is that psychotherapy is misunderstood. More specifically, the various schools of psychotherapy are based on normative conditions which describe the aims of psychotherapy (i.e., the 'ethos' of the psychotherapy schools). This is the topic of Chapter 5.

The policy statement for evidence-based practice in psychology is based on a specific kind of normative ethics. More precisely, it is based on utilitarianism. Nonetheless, this ethical foundation is not explicated in the policy statement. Consequently, it takes effect and shapes psychotherapy *implicitly*. It is important to uncover the ethics regulating psychotherapy practice to ask whether it is suitable to regulate a complex practice like psychotherapy. This will be addressed in Chapter 6.

Evidence-based practice in psychology was formulated as a tripartite concept (consisting of 'best available research,' 'clinical expertise,' and 'patient's characteristics, culture, and preferences'). The intention undergirding the tripartite structure was that the policy statement should incorporate more than scientific findings. However, the policy statement is conceptually inconsistent. It does not fulfil the ambition of being a tripartite concept. In its current form, evidence-based practice in psychology only consists of one component namely 'best available research.' Chapter 7 identifies some probable causes for why evidence-based practice in psychology failed to become a tripartite concept. It also provides some arguments for why it should be a tripartite concept.

One last question is how evidence-based practice in psychology can be developed into a principle that can regulate psychological practices (typically psychotherapy) more adequately. Evidence-based medicine has been revised continuously. A regulatory principle such as evidence-based practice in psychology should emanate from and reflect the distinctive character of psychotherapy. Integration is a key concept in the policy statement. The last objective of the book is to suggest improvements of evidence-based practice in psychology in light of the criticisms that has been presented throughout the book. This will be described in Chapter 8.

Chapter 9, which is the last chapter of the book, concludes the arguments that have been presented throughout the book. The main intention is to preserve the aspects that are valuable in evidence-based practice but also to summarise problematic aspects.

References

American Psychological Association. (2006). Presidential task force on evidence-based practice. *American Psychologist*, *61*, 271–285. http://doi.org/10.1037/0003-066X.61.4.271

Anderson, C. A., & Bushman, B. J. (2002). Human aggression. *Annual Review of Psychology*, *53*(1), 27–51. http://doi.org/10.1146/annurev.psych.53.100901.135231

Feyerabend, P. K. (2010). *Against method*. London: Verso Books.

Hacking, I. (1999). *The social construction of what?* Cambridge, MA: Harvard University Press.

Maturo, A. (2012). Medicalization: Current concept and future directions in a bionic society. *Mens Sana Monographs*, *10*(1), 122–133. http://doi.org/10.4103/0973-1229.91587

Moore, E. S. (2004). Children and the changing world of advertising. *Journal of Business Ethics*, *52*(2), 161–167. http://doi.org/10.1023/B:BUSI.0000035907.66617.f5

Nietzsche, F. (2012). *The genealogy of morals*. Newburyport: Dover Publications.

Popper, K. (1963). *Conjectures and refutations: The growth of scientific knowledge*. London: Routledge.

Popper, K. (2014). *The logic of scientific discovery*. Mansfield Centre, CT: Martino Publishing.

Ricoeur, P. (1970). *Freud & philosophy: An essay on interpretation*. New Haven, CT: Yale University Press.

Sellars, W. (1963). *Science, perception and reality*. New York, NY: Humanities Press.

2 Science, politics, and the technification of psychotherapy

Historical sources indicate that mental illness has been an integral part of human history. The Ebers Papyrus, which dates back to ancient Egyptian (appx 1500 BC), describes what we today call depression and dementia (Bryan, 1930). Another historical example is the Greek tragedies with protagonists experiencing trauma. A well-known character is Oedipus from Sophocles' (497–406 BC) plays. We can also find ancient descriptions of psychological pain in various religions. All the four noble truths in Buddhism are concerned with suffering (Gellner & Gombrich, 2015). Other historical accounts describe how societies in former historical eras have conceptualised mental illness. The 'Ships of Fools,' which travelled European waters in the Middle Ages and Renaissance, allegedly carried people with mental illness across the shores. It was assumed that the water had a healing effect and consequently that the contact with water could relieve their symptoms. In the subsequent historical era, called the Classical Period, people with mental illnesses were understood as 'beasts' in the sense that their mental illness stripped them of their humanity. Consequently, the most common ways of treating mental illnesses became brutish ('breaking in' patients like animals with the use of whips) (Foucault, 2001).

Historical descriptions of the understanding of mental illnesses should humble us. They serve as reminders that we living now (probably) have blind spots (Foucault, 2001). Like the example above, the example of drapetomania illustrates the point in a disturbing manner. Drapetomania, or the alleged 'fleeing disease,' was a diagnosis used to designate slaves who wanted to escape. To contemporaries these moral presuppositions are absurd as we believe that that no person should be kept as a slave. Thus, the slaves' wish to flee is nothing but legitimate. However, in the historical context in which drapetomania emerged, slavery was not only legitimate. The resistance against slavery was taken as an unmistaken sign of mental illness.

Fortunately, the current political context and cultural background from which we understand mental illness is different. Nonetheless, our

DOI: 10.4324/9781003512141-2

understanding also arises within a context which colours our conception of mental illness, as well as what constitutes a good life and a good society. It is not possible to understand what mental illness is or how we think about psychotherapy without taking this context into consideration. However, some deeply held current presuppositions will probably not be accepted by future generations. In this sense, history can make us intellectually humble through highlighting the fact that we are historical actors. Thus, we have a limited perspective. The best alternative is, then, to make use of various resources that may reveal problematic aspects of our understanding and treatment of mental illnesses.

Psychology: A pre-paradigmatic science?

We have been concerned with mental illnesses for quite some time. A big proportion of humanity is affected by it. In addition, there have been a drastic development in science and technology. Thus, it is perhaps somewhat surprising that we do not understand it better. The scientific understanding of 'natural phenomena' has become astonishing. The ability to produce technological innovations causes both excitement and concern (Jasanoff, 2016; Mitchell, 2019). At the same time, it is symptomatic of our culture that we tend to look to science and technology itself for solutions to problems caused by science and technology.

Different sciences have different levels of maturity. Some have well-established theories and methods with broad consensus. Others are more pluralistic and have several foundational issues. Psychology is often considered as the latter type of science. There simply is no general theoretical framework within psychology. Drawing on Thomas Kuhn's (1922–1996) nomenclature, psychology may be described as a 'pre-paradigmatic' science (Jackson, 2017; Kuhn, 2012; Melchert, 2016).

Some examples may illustrate the status quo. There is no established way of describing mental illnesses. Currently, descriptive diagnoses are dominating. Descriptive diagnoses are built on descriptions of clusters symptoms, typically without describing the aetiology (American Psychiatric Association, 2013; World Health Organization, 1992). According to Mayes and Horwitz (2005), the descriptive diagnostics were introduced as a scientific standardisation tool. They were not intended for use in clinical practice. The standardisation facilitates comparison of different scientific studies. Despite their intended use, descriptive diagnoses are currently being used as clinical tools.

The clinical value of descriptive diagnoses has been questioned. Allen Frances, who led the work developing Diagnostic and Statistical Manual of Mental Disorders DSM-IV, has criticised DSM-V (the subsequent version) harshly (Frances, 2013). This illustrates the uncertainty linked with psychiatric nosology. The discussions related to psychiatric diagnoses have been concerned with everything from the number of categories (Caspi et al., 2014), whether a classification based on biological and neuroscientific knowledge is more 'scientific' (Insel, 2014), and if 'the same' diagnosis has the same content and meaning in different cultures (Kirmayer, 1989; Kirmayer & Ryder, 2016). In short, a lot of work remains until a satisfactory psychiatric nosology is established.

Psychology consists of many different research methods. Several of these traditions are based on conflicting premises. Publications in scientific journals represent different theoretical traditions and quality criteria (Appelbaum et al., 2018; Levitt et al., 2018). In other words, there is theoretical and methodological pluralism in psychology.

In addition, there are several psychotherapy schools which differ markedly. Some estimates indicate that there are several hundred psychotherapy schools (Lambert, 2013). The American Psychological Association, however, distinguishes between five different main schools. These are behavioural psychology, cognitive psychology, psychoanalytic/psychodynamic psychology, humanistic-existential psychology, and eclectic/integrative approaches. There are significant differences between the schools, both with regard to epistemic and ethical questions (we will take a closer look at the latter in Chapter 5).

It is likely that the pluralism reflects characteristics of psychology and psychotherapy. The continuous revisions and fundamental discussions reflect the complexity of these objects. There are no signs that psychology will have a 'unifying' theory or theorist. Maybe, then, psychology is a non-paradigmatic science. A pre-paradigmatic science strives for unity. A non-paradigmatic science is pluralistic and incorporates a diversity of perspectives. Rather than reducing complexity to be able to draw simple and unambiguous conclusions, one can recognise and try to understand psychological phenomena in their complexity. In practice, the question is how much complexity regulative principles such as evidence-based practice in psychology can and should have. One of the main points of this book is that any regulation of psychotherapy must include ethics.

Modernity

Modernity is a term with many meanings. Here, modernity describes the transition to the renaissance in which science became a chief instrument for progress. One of its key thinkers is the French philosopher René Descartes (1596–1650). Descartes' most important philosophical project was to find an unambiguous foundation for knowledge. Through a sceptical method, Descartes hoped that he could identify something indubitably true. Descartes found the foundation in the fact that there must be something that is thinking (while doubting). This led to the famous phrase 'I think, therefore I am' (in Latin 'cogito ergo sum'). Descartes' most significant contribution to modern science was to refute radical scepticism and corroborating epistemology. In Descartes' (1998, 2017) epistemology, science ought to be mathematical and modelled on physics. This ideal has been influential in many sciences, including psychology (Michell, 2003).

Sir Francis Bacon (1561–1626) is another central modern philosopher (who lived prior to Descartes). Bacon is often regarded the founder of modern empirical science. His scientific method emphasised direct testing of empirical statements. Like Descartes, Bacon argued that epistemology must be critical. He argued that the human mind is a 'crooked mirror' that tends to misrepresent the world. Accordingly, scientific observations must be methodical to avoid typical human pitfalls and represent the world correctly (Bacon, 2000). Bacon's ideas have been central in the history of science, and it is an important backdrop for evidence-based practice (Cochrane, 1999; Solesbury, 2001).

Another central feature of modernity is the assumption that scientific knowledge will lead to progress. Francis Bacon's well-known slogan 'knowledge is power' reflects this optimism (Rodrígez García, 2001). Descartes' philosophy is also based on this presumption (Schouls, 1987). However, few philosophers reflect a belief in progress more clearly than the enlightenment philosopher Nicolas de Condorcet (1743–1794). In the text 'Outlines of an historical view of the progress of the human mind,' Condorcet (1795) wrote:

> [M]ay it not be expected that the human race will be meliorated by new discoveries in the sciences and the arts, and, as an unavoidable consequence, in the means of individual and general prosperity; by farther progress in the principles of conduct, and in moral practice; and lastly, by the real improvement of our faculties, moral, intellectual and physical, which may be the result either of the improvement of the instruments which increase the power and direct the exercise of those faculties, or of the improvement of our natural organization itself?
>
> (p. 251)

According to Condorcet, science will result in radical improvements in political institutions and, more dramatically, in humanity itself. Today, a similar belief exists among transhumanists. Transhumanism is an ideology seeking to transcend the natural limitations of humanity prior to the development of modern technology (Bostrom, 2011). Examples of such improvements are technological changes in the human genetic material (e.g., through CRISPR-Cas-9) (Doudna & Charpentier, 2014) or to insert electronic devices directly into the human body or brain. Condorcet's (1795) quote also reflects a vehement belief in the power of change through political reform. This does in turn reflect a belief that we (to a great extent) can predict the consequences of different political resolutions – a premise that is highly questionable (Bauman, 2000; Scott, 2020).

The tenets of modernity have been criticised. A well-known critic is the French philosopher Jean-François Lyotard (1924–1998). Lyotard wrote a knowledge report in the middle of the second half of the 20th century. Lyotard (1979) claimed that we, living centuries after the modern philosophers, have reasons to question the tenets of modernity. We do not believe that science provides *necessarily* true knowledge about the world. Nor do we believe that science necessarily leads to progress for humanity. Lyotard's point is not that science is without epistemic or practical value. His point is that we must be more subtle in thinking about science and its limitations. In 'the postmodern condition', we have moved away from *presupposing* that an epistemic foundation can provide universal knowledge and progress. Instead, science and its consequences must be analysed in detail. This is described as a transition from grand narratives (e.g., 'science reveals true and useful propositions about the world') to small narratives (e.g., 'which premises do knowledge rest on in a specific context, and what are the associated advantages and disadvantages?') (Lyotard, 1979).

Luckily, the quality of science is evaluated regularly. One way to examine scientific quality is to investigate whether scientists follow the scientific norms. A central scientific norm (particularly important in the natural sciences) is objectivity (Merton, 1973). Here, objectivity means that researchers are not prejudiced and prefer a certain outcome when they test propositions. Nonetheless, scientific journals have preferred positive results that 'verify' hypotheses. This practice has the designation publication bias (DeVito & Goldacre, 2019). Publication bias sometimes motivates researchers to adjust data collection and/or the statistical analyses (to confirm the hypotheses). This practice is called p-hacking (Head, Holman, Lanfear, Kahn, & Jennions, 2015). Based on a suspicion that scientific practices may threaten the credibility of science, the statistician John P.A. Ioannidis conducted a meta-statistical analysis. The published article got the title *Why most published research findings are false*. Ioannidis argued that there is reason to believe that most scientific conclusions in healthcare sciences are false (Ioannidis, 2005). The background is a combination of unreliable research practices and the inherent vulnerability of probabilistic methods (e.g., type I and II errors). In other words, Ioannidis' publication indicates that there is a big gap between the epistemic tenet of modernity and today's scientific standards and practices.

Another way to test scientific quality is through large-scale replications. In a project called Open Science Collaboration, Brian Nosek and colleagues tested whether psychological findings could be replicated. They analysed 100 research articles published in three esteemed peer-reviewed journals. Originally, 97% of the studies showed statistically significant results. In the replications, only 36% got the same result. The palpable gap led to the designation 'replication crisis.' As the original findings could not be replicated in additional attempts, a number of psychological theories have also been questioned or revised (Jarret, 2016).

In the sciences where empirical results are more consistent, modernity's second premise remains problematic (i.e., science entails progress). Let's take a 'hard science' such as physics as an example. Physics has not exclusively led to human progress. Not only has knowledge from physics been used to develop the nuclear bomb, the role of 'the hard sciences' in the industrial revolution as well as in the current climate crisis also makes this premise unreliable. We cannot presuppose the goodness of science; we must identify advantages and disadvantages in a case-by-case manner.

Scientific quantification

The belief in quantification as an epistemic tool dates further back than Ancient Greece. Plato (427–347 BC) considered numerical knowledge to be eternally true (Michell, 2003; Plato, 1993, 2010). Quantification also played an important part in the scientific revolution. Many of the philosophers of the scientific revolution proposed a numerical foundation for science. Galileo Galilei (1564–1642) is a good example. In his philosophical writings, Galilei distinguished between primary and secondary sensory qualities. Primary sensory qualities belong to nature itself and are mathematical and geometrical. The secondary sensory qualities are nature as it appears to humans through their sensory apparatus. According to Galilei, only primary qualities exist. Thus, mathematics and geometry are the only means to understand the world the way it is:

> Philosophy is written in this grand book, the universe, which stands continually open to our gaze. But the book cannot be understood unless one first learns to comprehend the language and read the letters in which it is composed. It is written in the language of mathematics, and its characters are triangles, circles, and other geometric figures without which it is humanly impossible to understand a single word of it; without these, one wanders about in a dark labyrinth.
>
> (Galilei, 1623, p. 4)

The idea that we need to use mathematics (and geometry) to understand the world has, however, been criticised. Edmund Husserl (1838–1917) criticised Galilei (and the other philosophers from the scientific revolution) for conflating scientific methods and scientific presuppositions. Husserl identified some pre-scientific conditions of possibility. These pre-scientific conditions of possibility are necessary to understand any phenomenon, including the objects of science. Husserl coins the pre-scientific conditions of possibility the 'lifeworld.' The 'lifeworld' originates from our everyday practices (Husserl, 1970). We know what mountains, anger, and 'rosy red' are, because we have encountered these phenomena in everyday life. Science and technology make it possible to reduce the mountain to minerals, to operationalise anger as 'intended physical damage to objects, other persons or oneself,' and to give 'rosy red' an oscillation number. This, however, does not make the 'lifeworld' less primordial. When researchers are investigating scientific objects, they rely on an understanding existing before the scientific investigation (hence the designation 'conditions of possibility'). The scientific object of inquiry is not the phenomenon as it exists in its natural context. Rather, it is a partial and reduced version of the phenomenon (often in a controlled context). The natural phenomenon is part of a complex web of meaning which constitutes the world as we understand it. This does not only apply to the scientific object in isolation, but also other aspects that it is necessary to know something about to be able to carry out a scientific investigation. This includes linguistic competency, how to use research tools, and social norms.

Ideally, science helps us understand phenomena better. However, sometimes it can in fact worsen our understanding and practices. An example of the latter is behaviouristic expert advice on parenting in the 20th century. Behaviourism reflects an epistemological position coined radical empiricism (Benjamin, 2014). Radical empiricism entails basing knowledge claims solely on experience (typically qua empirical science). Some behaviourists argued that you should treat your children as miniature adults (Bigelow & Morris, 2001). J.B. Watson (1878–1958) and R.R. Watson (1898–1835) gave the following advice to parents

> Let your behaviour always be objective and kindly firm. Never hug and kiss them, never let them sit in your lap. If you must, kiss them once on the forehead when they say good night. Shake hands with them in the morning. Give them a pat on the head if they have made an extraordinarily good job of a difficult task.
>
> (1928, p. 73)

Today, most people will deem this advice outlandish. Of course, the scientific standards were different from today's standards. However, the main point is the relation between scientific knowledge and the 'lifeworld.' According to Fass (2016), Watson and Watson's advice conflicted with an American tradition where maternal care and patience were well-established ideals. Thus, the parents who chose to follow Watson and Watson's advice did so because they wanted to have a scientifically informed parenting style (Fass, 2016). The example illustrates that science does not come with a guarantee to provide us with good advice or lead to better life conditions. This implies that we also need analytical resources to assess science critically (to optimise its utility).

A significant part of (quantitative) sciences is today probabilistic (Kitcher, 2009). Statistical methods are used to find out the probability of a proposition or inference being true. The probability is expressed using numbers. However, with probabilism comes the potential for misuse (Oreskes & Conway, 2010; Porter, 1995). Oreskes and Conway (2010) have shown that numbers can be used as a means of persuasion. They are particularly potent in sciences with complex objects of inquiries. Numbers have been used to undermine that 'smoking increases the probability of cancer' and 'human actions contribute towards climate changes.' Oreskes and Conway (2010) also show the great impact that numerical argumentation can have in institutions like the court of law. This poses a potential problem in psychology, which often analyses complex objects of inquiry. Of course, numbers can be very useful. They are less polysemous than words. To fulfil its potential, however, quantitative science must meet the same critical standards as other scientific claims.

Positivism

Ever since the Pre-Socratic philosophers, scholars have had an ambition of giving precise descriptions of the world (Howatson, 2011). For a long time, this was the task of philosophy. As several sciences such as physics, biology, and psychology emerged, some understood the relationship between philosophy and the special sciences as a division of labour. The sciences describe 'how the world is like.' Philosophy deals with the overarching questions of truth, knowledge, and ethics. This tendency was particularly prominent in the 19th century in which many new scientific disciplines emerged.

Auguste Comte (1798–1857) has given an influential epistemological basis for many sciences (Martineau, 1896). Comte's epistemology partly reflects the thinking of German philosopher G.W.F. Hegel (1770–1831). Hegel claimed that the history of the West consisted of different epochs. One historical epoch is superseded by a new epoch where tensions permeating the previous era are overcome. Comte's epistemology is based on a similar theory of historical stages and progress. According to Comte, 19th-century science had rendered the preceding theological and metaphysical phases obsolete. Whereas the theological phase was dominated by myths (e.g., religion), the metaphysical phase in which knowledge was speculative and non-empirical (e.g., philosophy). The scientific stage, in contrast, knowledge means empirical knowledge. Comte refers to empirical knowledge as positive knowledge (hence, the term positivism). Comte claimed that all domains (including humans and society) should be subject to scientific analyses. The ultimate aim, however, was social reform to benefit all layers of society. In other words, Comte's positivism has political aims (Comte, 1908).

Comte's epistemology also includes a science hierarchy. It is built on a principle that there is a reverse proportional relationship between complexity and generalisability. The least complex sciences (e.g., physics) have the highest generalisability. The most complex sciences (e.g., sociology) have the lowest generalisability. In Comte's hierarchy, today's psychology would probably have been classified as a very complex science with low generalisability (Martineau, 1896). One important implication is that scientific findings have to be adjusted in practical use. Scientific knowledge about psychological phenomena needs practical translation.

Psychology was established as a scientific discipline in the 19th century. It is often linked to Wilhelm Wundt's (1832–1920) experimental psychology at the University of Leipzig in 1879. However, Wundt's theory of science is sometimes misrepresented. Wundt argued that non-experimental research should be a part of academic psychology. Scientific questions not susceptible to experimental psychology should be part of a folk psychology (in German 'Volkerpsychologie'). Folk psychology was supposed to be a qualitative supplement to experimental psychology. In other words, Wundt saw clear limitations in experimental psychology, a point that has not been communicated adequately throughout the history of psychology (Hergenhahn, 2001).

There is a reason to question the historical progressivism in positivistic philosophy. Neither the political, financial, nor ecological spheres progress steadily. In psychology, neither the psychological concepts, methods, nor theories are *necessarily* improving with time. Marginalised theories, methods, and concepts may re-enter the mainstream of psychological research (Lakatos, 1978; Laudan, 1977). There may also be valuable insights from previous historical eras or other cultures that render this assumption problematic. Some argues that the understanding of mental illness in the Renaissance was more humane than in the subsequent classical era. Nor does empirical knowledge render philosophical knowledge obsolete. Conceptual and theoretical understanding is necessary to develop empirical sciences. Foundational questions and premises do not dissipate because researchers and practitioners pay them less attention.

Logical positivism

Logical positivism (or logical empiricism) is linked to the Vienna Circle. The Vienna Circle was a group of intellectuals who met regularly in the interwar period under Moritz Schlick's (1882–1936) leadership (Ayer, 1959). The main purpose of the gatherings was to find a rigorous foundation for science (Sigmund, 2017). The Austrian philosopher Ludwig Wittgenstein (1889–1951) and his Tractatus Logico-Philosophicus was a major source of inspiration (Ayer, 1959; Wittgenstein, 2001). The Vienna Circle interpretation of the Tractatus was as follows. There are only two types of meaningful statements. Analytical statements are concerned with the relation between terms. To understand the term 'bachelor', it suffices to know the meaning of 'an unmarried man.' In other words, empirical investigations are irrelevant to understand the meaning terms like 'bachelor.' Synthetic statements are empirical propositions. To say anything about how the world is like, we must observe it. The logical positivists claimed that the meaning of statements about the world is inseparably linked with how they can be observed. This is known as their 'principle of verification.' Echoing Hume (2009), the logical positivists argued that nothing but analytic and synthetic statements are meaningful (Ayer, 1936).

The logical positivist doctrine influences the conception of ethics. An ethical theory associated with logical positivism is called emotivism. According to emotivism, the normative part of language is non-observable and thus not meaningful. Normative statements are nothing more than an expression of emotions. If somebody claims that 'it is wrong to kill,' they might just as well have exclaimed 'boo, murder!'. This affects the relationship between ethics and science. In general, emotivism entails that normativity (being nonsensical) is absolute distinct from empirical investigations. Science describes the world (full stop). A.J. Ayer (1910–1989), one of the most prominent spokesmen of logical positivism, wrote:

> […] in so far as statements of value are significant, they are ordinary 'scientific' statements; and that in so far as they are not scientific, they are not in the literal sense significant, but are simply expressions of emotion which can be neither true nor false.
>
> (1936, p. 64)

Logical positivism is sometimes characterised as scientistic. Scientism is the belief that science should have unrestricted authority in all questions (Sorell, 2013). Tjeltveit (1999) has introduced a useful distinction between philosophical scientism and de facto scientism. Philosophical scientism tries to show why science should have unlimited authority. Some take the logical positivists to represent philosophical scientism. De facto scientism, on the other hand, simply accepts that science should have unlimited authority, without providing any arguments for this stance. De facto scientism is a conventionalism that exist among some researchers (and practitioners). In psychology, like in other disciplines, scientific legitimacy can be crucial. According to Tjeltveit this has sometimes resulted in attempts to rid psychology of 'philosophical' thinking. Some psychologists (like B.F. Skinner) were philosophically informed scientists. Yet, over some generations, philosophical scientism has turned into de facto scientism. As such (de facto) scientism, which informs certain parts of psychology, is not justified by its proponents (Tjeltveit, 1999).

In 1967, logical positivism was described as 'dead, or as dead as a philosophical movement ever becomes' (Passmore, 1967, p. 57). Nonetheless, logical positivism still influences parts of science and the understanding of science. One consequence is the sustenance of the artificial divide between facts and values. In psychology and psychotherapy, de facto scientism deteriorates the understanding and regulation of practice. In psychotherapy, facts and values are deeply integrated. Consequently, an improved conceptualisation of psychotherapy is needed (Berg & Slaattelid, 2017).

Bureaucratisation

Bureaucracy describes forms of administration and management, typically in the public sector. Bureaucracies implement the decisions of those in power through various types of governing bodies such as the elected representatives in a democracy or the board in an organisation (Poulin, 2013). The sociologist Max Weber (1864–1920) provided an analysis of bureaucracies. The most influential types emerged within modern European states. Weber claimed that bureaucracies are characterised by some relatively distinct areas of competence with allocated rights and obligations, held by staff with relevant qualifications. These undertake their responsibilities according to the rules and in an impersonal manner. The more efficient the bureaucracy is, the less it matters who the bureaucrats and the subjects are.

However, the bureaucratic rules may be formulated more or less abstractly. Abstract rules incorporate more diversity. An example of a relatively abstract rule could be 'Health services (e.g., psychotherapeutic practice) should be based on a specific type of evidence (e.g., randomised controlled trials).' If this rule applies universally, all psychotherapists must utilise treatment methods tested by randomised controlled trials. Bureaucratic rules can, moreover, dictate practices in great detail. One example is when psychotherapists use highly standardised treatment forms specifying the steps of treatment (similar to an algorithm). The bureaucratic ideal is that all cases that the bureaucracy defines as the same must be treated alike. This is known as the formal principle of equity formulated by Aristotle (2009).

Weber compares modern bureaucracies with administrative practices and ideals that were informal and largely nepotistic. Comparably, impersonal bureaucracies are very efficient with regard to both quality and cost-effectiveness. Bureaucracies serve a standardising function and secure more equal rights. This is relevant for the treatment of mental illness. In principle, patients should expect the same quality of treatment regardless of who they are. While, of course, in practice psychotherapists are more or less skilled (Hill & Castonguay, 2017). There are clear-cut examples of an unwanted variation in the healthcare service. One example is that people with a high socioeconomic status receive better healthcare service than people with a lower socioeconomic status (Lopes, Ravesteijn, Van Ourti, & Riuma llo-Herl, 2023). By the same token, some practices cannot be regulated in detail. The question is how much individual variation should be permitted. If there is a high degree of relevant individual variation, bureaucratisation run the risk of reducing the quality of services. If patients have different treatment needs, a strict and general regulation might reduce the quality of treatment. Psychiatric diagnoses contain a high degree of within category variation. In other words, two patients with the same diagnosis can have very different treatment needs. Consequently, it is important to regulate practices like psychotherapy to incorporate relevant individual differences.

Standardisation

Sociologists Timmermans and Berg (2003) claimed that one of the most important features of modern Western cultures is the establishment of standards. They distinguished between four different types of standards. Design standards are the description of individual components in systems that ensures equality and compatibility. Design standards can be anything from technical requirements for offices to the duration of consultations. The second type is terminological standards. One example of a terminological standard is diagnosis manuals cataloguing mental disorders. A third type is performance standards establishing the aims for an activity. The performance standard could be symptom reduction or enhancing the ability to work through psychotherapeutic treatment. The fourth type is procedural standards, which describe steps or elements in an activity. An example could be highly standardised psychotherapeutic treatments which specify the elements of therapy.

Timmermans and Berg (2003) analysed evidence-based medicine. Thus, it is relevant for evidence-based practice in psychology. Standardising is at the heart of evidence-based practice in psychology. The most relevant question is how these standards impact the quality of the services. One of the most important indicators of high quality will be the performance standards. Universal performance standards are difficult to develop in psychotherapy because many individual factors need to be taken into consideration. Simplistic performance standards will obstruct the quality of treatment.

New public management

New public management is a term emanating from academic analyses of the reforms in public sector in the 1970s and 1980s (Gruening, 2001). The background for the reforms was economic recession and several large tax rebellions. In new public management (public), services are governed as private sector. Some key principles are open competition and goal-oriented management. The goal-oriented management economically incentivises goal attainment. One example could be that a completed (or successful) psychotherapeutic treatment results in economic reimbursements. These managerial principles presumably result in cost-effective services which ultimately benefit the population. New public management institutions such as hospitals and schools are run like businesses, and the users are consumers. Service users' freedom of choice presumably lead to high-quality services. One explanation for the emergence of new public management in the healthcare sector is the increasing expenses. Healthcare is the largest expenditure in many Western countries. This is also the case in countries where a large part of the health sector is privatised (Organisation for Economic Co-operation and Development, 2019).

Two central features of new public management are often forgotten. The first is the idea that administration and politics are separated. Administration is understood as politically 'neutral.' The second is that 'new public management' is linked to an increased use of information technology. National health services use various information technology devices in the hope of increasing the efficiency of the services and reducing government costs (Gruening, 2001).

The idea that the administration is politically neutral is disputed. In practice, political neutrality often entails implicit political ideals. For this reason, it is important to explore the ideals of allegedly neutral political actors. This is pivotal to improve political ideals or practices. The reason for introducing information technology is normally that it will lead to more efficient services. At the same time, the use of information technology raises new problems. One example is whether services that are delivered by use of information technology and human-beings are compatible. This question will be raised in Chapter 6.

Professions

In a fictional Chinese taxonomy authored by Jorge Luis Borges (1899–1986), we find categories such as:

- The animals belonging to the emperor.
- The animals drawn with a very fine camelhair brush.
- The animals that from a long way off look like flies.

The taxonomy is a reminder that the way we perceive the world depends on our categories. Most categories are contingent and, thus, subject to change (Borges, 1993). This is also true with regard to the demarcation of professions. Psychology encompass the humanities, social science, and natural science. More precisely it merges with disciplines such as philosophy, sociology, biology, and medicine. Within a science there is an ongoing battle for legitimacy. The history of psychology is full of examples of schools battling for legitimacy and hegemony. The policy statement for evidence-based practice in psychology may be seen as part of such a polemic. Anticipating future developments, the policy statement will probably change in light of (counter)arguments. No ideal – and certainly no ideal based on scientific evidence – should be exempted from academic critique.

While there may be tensions within different fields, such tensions are often more pronounced between professions. The mandate of a professions is not given, and they compete for legitimacy. There is an important distinction between professions that have a scientific foundation and those that do not. For science-based professions, science has become important for whether governments and users trust services. The professions with the best results increase their share of 'the market' (e.g., 'the health market'). If research suggests that psychological treatments are (as or) more efficient than medical treatments, politicians typically allocate more funds to psychological treatments and vice versa. This entails that any profession must make strategic choices in relation to adjacent professions. Medicine is particularly relevant for psychotherapy. Medicine has been instrumental in the orientation of clinical psychology. Nonetheless, there are some fundamental differences between the two practices. While strategic considerations play a part, an unrestricted strategical thinking could reduce the legitimacy of a practice like psychotherapy in the longer run. One of the main arguments in this book is that evidence-based practice in psychology is unbalanced in favour of strategic considerations. It is necessary to reform the regulatory principles to get in touch with the nature of psychotherapy.

Technification of psychotherapy

It is very difficult to predict the effects of technology. Thus, almost by necessity, critical analyses of technology are speculative. For this reason, fiction can be a good source for critical thinking about technology as this genre is less rule-governed than scientific texts or other non-fiction genres. There are several classical examples of fictional literature analysing technology. Some examples are H.G. Wells' (1866–1946) 'The Island of Dr. Moreau' (Wells, 2017), Philip K. Dick's (1928–1982) 'Do Androids Dream of Electric Sheep?' (Dick, 1968), and Mary Shelley's (1797–1851) 'Frankenstein' (Shelley, 2001). In the novel 'Frankenstein,' we meet the young scientist, Victor Frankenstein. Frankenstein has just lost his mother and devotes himself to science and technology to deal with the grief. Frankenstein creates a living being, but the creature turns out to be a monster that causes fear and disgust. In despair of not fitting into the human world, the monster gives his creator (Victor Frankenstein) an ultimatum. If Frankenstein does not create another creature/monster, he threatens to kill his family. In fear of the damage a new monster may cause, Frankenstein chooses not to make a new monster. Consequently, his monster kills several of his family members (Shelley, 2001).

This story is a warning against hubris. Victor Frankenstein has the technical knowledge and skill to create a monster. However, he lacks the wisdom to abstain from doing it. The creation of his monster is motivated by intense grief due to the loss of his mother. This may reflect the vulnerability and pain our uncontrolled destinies cause. When Frankenstein, once bitten twice shy, chooses not to create a new monster, this may indicate that he chooses not to solve problems caused by technology with new technology. The fundamental acknowledgement is the difficulty of predicting the effects of (new) technology.

The narrative structure of the novel is also interesting. The story is told through letters which captain Robert Walton writes to his sister, Margaret Walton Saville, who presents the story to the reader. Robert Walton meets Victor Frankenstein at the North Pole where the latter has just failed to capture the monster. Walton writes down his story. This reflects *how hard* predicting problematic aspects of technology and science is. We are forced to see the limitations of science and technology through several narrative filters. This problematising of the story's credibility is a central part of the novel's criticism of technology (Shelley, 2001).

There is no *necessary* connection between technology and evidence-based practice in psychology. However, there is a strong connection between science and technology. Scientific evidence is at the very heart of evidence-based practice in psychology. At a minimum, this invites a technification of psychotherapy. Technology is a description of means that are suitable for achieving certain ends. It reflects how evidence-based practice in psychology regulates psychotherapy. Evidence-based practice in psychology is (first and foremost) a principle for evaluating the efficiency of means. However, technification of psychotherapy makes us less capable of evaluating whether its ends are desirable. Technology often presupposes that its aims are indisputably good. In psychotherapy, there are few (if any) ends which do not need to be related to a certain context. Thus, practical wisdom and ethical discretion must be an essential part of psychotherapy.

Conclusion

Naturally, the ideas that have been presented in this chapter do not exhaust the backdrop for evidence-based practice in psychology. Neither do the traditions harmonise perfectly. Nonetheless, the traditions are related. The modern and positivistic conception of science fits bureaucracies and establishing standards. New public management is often based on scientific analyses of efficiency and within established bureaucratic structures. The fact and value distinction found in logical positivism may serve to corroborate the idea of a value-free administration in new public management. The struggle between professions takes place in market economies that reflect features of new public management, often with scientific findings as a legitimising tool. The technification of psychotherapy is closely linked to both bureaucratisation which standardises the targets for the activity and the understanding of scientific analyses which reduces psychotherapy to a pure means. Together, these traditions may guide the thinking related to psychotherapy in a manner which naturalises these ideals. As we have seen, all these traditions have problems hindering a sound regulation of psychotherapy. Actually, they contribute to a limited conceptualisation of psychotherapy. As we shall see, however, there are both academic and practical arguments that show how these traditions attenuate the understanding of psychotherapy.

References

American Psychiatric Association. (2013). *Diagnostic and statistical manual of mental disorders: DSM-5* (5th ed.). Washington, DC: American Psychiatric Association.

Appelbaum, M., Cooper, H., Kline, R. B., Mayo-Wilson, E., Nezu, A. M., & Rao, S. M. (2018). Journal article reporting standards for quantitative research in psychology: The APA Publications and Communications Board task force report. *American Psychologist*, *73*(1), 3–25. https://doi.org/10.1037/amp0000191

Aristotle. (2009). *The Nicomachean ethics* (D. Ross & L. Brown, Trans.). Oxford: Oxford University Press.

Ayer, A. J. (1936). *Language, truth and logic*. London: Penguin books.

Ayer, A. J. (1959). Editor's introduction. In A. J. Ayer (Ed.), *Logical positivism* (pp. 3–28). New York, NY: Free Press.

Bacon, F. (2000). *The new organon*. Cambridge: Cambridge University Press.

Bauman, Z. (2000). *Liquid modernity*. Cambridge: Polity Press.

Benjamin, L. T. (2014). *A brief history of modern psychology* (2nd ed.). Hoboken, NJ: Wiley.

Berg, H., & Slaattelid, R. (2017). Facts and values in psychotherapy: A critique of the empirical reduction of psychotherapy within evidence-based practice. *Journal of Evaluation in Clinical Practice*, *23*(5), 1075–1080. https://doi.org/10.1111/jep.12739

Bigelow, K. M., & Morris, E. K. (2001). John B. Watson's advice on child rearing: Some historical context. *Behavioral Development Bulletin*, *10*(1), 26–30. https://doi.org/10.1037/h0100479

Borges, J. L. (1993). The analytical language of John Wilkins. In Jorge Luis Borges & Ruth L. C. Simms (Eds.), *Other inquisitions*. Austin, TX: University of Texas Press.

Bostrom, N. (2011). A history of transhumanist thought. In M. Rectenwald & L. Carl (Eds.), *Academic writing across the disciplines* (pp. 1–25). New York, NY: Pearson Longman.

Bryan, C. P. (1930). *Ancient Egyptian medicine: The Ebers papyrus*. London: Ares Publishers.

Caspi, A., Houts, R. M., Belsky, D. W., Goldman-Mellor, S. J., Harrington, H., Israel, S., … Moffitt, T. E. (2014). The p factor: One general psychopathology factor in the structure of psychiatric disorders? *Clinical Psychological Science*, *2*(2), 119–137. https://doi.org/10.1177/2167702613497473

Cochrane, A. L. (1999). *Effectiveness and efficiency: Random reflections on health services*. London: Royal Society of Medicine Press.

Comte, A. (1908). *A general view of positivism*. London: George Routledge & Sons limited.

Condorcet, M. D. (1795). Outlines of an historical view of the progress of the human mind. Retrieved from https://oll.libertyfund.org/titles/condorcet-outlines-of-an-historical-view-of-the-progress-of-the-human-mind

Descartes, R. (1998). *A discourse on method and Meditations on first philosophy* (D. A. Cress, Trans. 4th ed.). Indianapolis, IN: Hacket Publishing Company.

Descartes, R. (2017). Principles of philosophy. Retrieved from http://www.earlymoderntexts.com/assets/pdfs/descartes1644part1.pdf

DeVito, N. J., & Goldacre, B. (2019). Catalogue of bias: Publication bias. *British Medical Journal: Evidence-Based Medicine*, *24*(2), 53–54. https://doi.org/10.1136/bmjebm-2018-111107

Dick, P. K. (1968). *Do androids dream of electric sheep?* New York, NY: Del Rey.

Doudna, J. A., & Charpentier, E. (2014). The new frontier of genome engineering with CRISPR-Cas9. *Science*, *346*(6213), 1258096. https://doi.org/10.1126/science.1258096

Fass, P. S. (2016). *The end of American childhood: A history of parenting from life on the frontier to the managed child*. Princeton, NJ: Princeton University Press.

Foucault, M. (2001). *Madness and civilization: A history of insanity in the age of reason*. London: Routledge.

Frances, A. (2013). The new crisis of confidence in psychiatric diagnosis. *Annals of Internal Medicine*, *159*(3), 221–222. https://doi.org/10.7326/0003-4819-159-3-201308060-00655

Galilei, G. (1623). The Assayer. In S. Drake (Ed.), *Discoveries and Opinions of Galileo* (pp. 237–238). New York: Knopf Doubleday Publishing Group.

Gellner, D. N., & Gombrich, R. (2015). Buddhism. In J. D. Wright (Ed.), *International encyclopedia of the social & behavioral sciences* (pp. 886–893). Oxford: Elsevier.

Gruening, G. (2001). Origin and theoretical basis of new public management. *International Public Management Journal*, *4*(1), 1–25. https://doi.org/10.1016/S1096-7494(01)00041-1

Head, M. L., Holman, L., Lanfear, R., Kahn, A. T., & Jennions, M. D. (2015). The extent and consequences of p-hacking in science. *PLoS Biology*, *13*(3), 1–15. http://doi.org/10.1371/journal.pbio.1002106

Hergenhahn, B. R. (2001). *An introduction to the history of psychology* (4th ed.). Belmont, CA: Wadsworth Thomson Learning.

Hill, C. E., & Castonguay, L. G. (2017). Therapist effects: Integration and conclusions. In L. G. Castonguay & C. E. Hill (Eds.), *How and why are some therapists better than others?: Understanding therapist effects* (pp. 325–341). Washington, DC: American Psychological Association.

Howatson, M. C. (2011). *The Oxford companion to classical literature* (3rd ed.). https://doi.org/10.1093/acref/9780199548545.001.0001

Hume, D. (2009). *A treatise of human nature: Being an attempt to introduce the experimental method of reasoning into moral subjects*. Auckland: The Floating Press.

Husserl, E. (1970). *The crisis of European sciences and transcendental phenomenology: An introduction to phenomenological philosophy*. Evanston, IL: Northwestern University Press.

Insel, T. R. (2014). The NIMH research domain criteria (RDoC) project: Precision medicine for psychiatry. *American Journal of Psychiatry*, *171*(4), 395–397. https://doi.org/10.1176/appi.ajp.2014.14020138

Ioannidis, J. P. A. (2005). Why most published research findings are false. *PLoS Medicine*, *2*(8), e124. https://doi.org/10.1371/journal.pmed.0020124

Jackson, M. R. (2017). Unified clinical science, or paradigm diversity?: Comment on Melchert. *American Psychologist*, *72*(4), 395–396. https://doi.org/10.1037/amp0000125

Jarret, C. (2016). Ten famous psychology findings that it's been difficult to replicate. *Research Digest*. Retrieved from https://digest.bps.org.uk/2016/09/16/ten-famous-psychology-findings-that-its-been-difficult-to-replicate/

Jasanoff, S. (2016). *The ethics of invention: Technology and the human future*. New York, NY: W. W. Norton & Company.

Kirmayer, L. J. (1989). Cultural variations in the response to psychiatric disorders and emotional distress. *Social Science and Medicine*, *29*(3), 327–339. https://doi.org/10.1016/0277-9536(89)90281-5

Kirmayer, L. J., & Ryder, A. G. (2016). Culture and psychopathology. *Current Opinion in Psychology*, *8*, 143–148. https://doi.org/10.1016/j.copsyc.2015.10.020

Kitcher, P. (2009). Scientific knowledge. In P. K. Moser (Ed.), *The Oxford handbook of epistemology*. https://doi.org/10.1093/oxfordhb/9780195301700.003.0014

Kuhn, T. (2012). *The structure of scientific revolutions* (4th ed.). Chicago, IL: University of Chicago Press.

Lakatos, I. (1978). *The methodology of scientific research programmes* (Vol. 1). New York, NY: Cambridge University Press.

Lambert, M. J. (2013). Introduction and historical overview. In M. J. Lambert (Ed.), *Bergin and Garfield's handbook of psychotherapy and behaviour change* (6th ed., pp. 3–20). Hoboken, NJ: John Wiley & Sons.

Laudan, L. (1977). *Progress and problems: Towards a theory of scientific growth*. Los Angeles, CA: University of California Press.

Levitt, H. M., Bamberg, M., Creswell, J. W., Frost, D. M., Josselson, R., & Suárez-Orozco, C. (2018). Journal article reporting standards for qualitative primary, qualitative meta-analytic, and mixed methods research in psychology: The APA Publications and Communications Board task force report. *American Psychologist*, *73*(1). https://doi.org/10.1037/amp0000151

Lopes, F. V., Ravesteijn, B., Van Ourti, T., & Riumallo-Herl, C. (2023). Income inequalities beyond access to mental health care: a Dutch nationwide record-linkage cohort study of baseline disease severity, treatment intensity, and mental health outcomes. *The Lancet Psychiatry*, *10*(8), 588–597. https://doi.org/10.1016/S2215-0366(23)00155-4

Lyotard, J.-F. (1979). *The postmodern condition: A report on knowledge*. Minneapolis, MN: University of Minnesota Press.

Martineau, H. (1896). *The positive philosophy of Auguste Comte* (Vol. I). London: George Bell & Sons.

Mayes, R., & Horwitz, A. V. (2005). DSM-III and the revolution in the classification of mental illness. *Journal of the History of the Behavioral Sciences*, *41*(3), 249–267. https://doi.org/10.1002/jhbs.20103

Melchert, T. P. (2016). Leaving behind our preparadigmatic past: Professional psychology as a unified clinical science. *American Psychologist*, *71*(6), 486–496. https://doi.org/10.1037/a004022

Merton, R. K. (1973). The normative structure of science. In R. K. Merton (Ed.), *The sociology of science: Theoretical and empirical investigations*. Chicago, IL: University of Chicago Press.

Michell, J. (2003). The quantitative imperative: Positivism, naive realism and the place of qualitative methods in psychology. *Theory & Psychology*, *13*(1), 5–31. https://doi.org/10.1177/0959354303013001758

Mitchell, M. (2019). *Artificial intelligence: A guide for thinking humans*. New York, NY: Farrar, Strauss and Giroux.

Oreskes, N., & Conway, E. M. (2010). *Merchants of doubt: How a handful of scientists obscured the truth on issues from tobacco smoke to global warming*. New York, NY: Bloomsbury Press.

Organisation for Economic Co-operation and Development. (2019). Health expenditure and financing. Retrieved from https://stats.oecd.org/Index.aspx?ThemeTreeId=9

Passmore, J. (1967). Logical Positivism. In P. Edwards (Ed.), *The encyclopedia of philosophy* (Vol. 5, pp. 52–57). New York, NY: Macmillan.

Plato. (1993). *The Republic*. New York, NY: Oxford University Press.

Plato. (2010). *Meno & Phaedo*. Cambridge: Cambridge University Press,

Porter, T. (1995). *Trust in numbers*. Princeton, NJ: Princeton University Press.

Poulin, T. E. (2013). Bureaucracy. In K. B. Penuel, M. Statler, & R. Hagen (Eds.), *Encyclopedia of crisis management*. https://doi.org/10.4135/9781452275956

Rodrígez García, J. M. (2001). Scientia potestas est – knowledge is power: Francis Bacon to Michel Foucault. *Neohelicon*, *28*(1), 109–121. https://doi.org/10.1023/A:1011901104984

Schouls, P. (1987). Descartes and the Idea of Progress. *History of Philosophy Quarterly*, *4*(4), 423–433. Retrieved from http://www.jstor.org/stable/27743829

Scott, J. C. (2020). *Seeing like a state: How certain schemes to improve the human condition have failed*. New Haven: Yale University Press.

Shelley, M. W. (2001). *Frankenstein*. New York, NY: Dover Publications.

Sigmund, K. (2017). *Exact thinking in demented times: The Vienna circle and the epic quest for the foundations of science*. New York, NY: Basic Books.

Solesbury, W. (2001). Evidence based policy: Whence it came and where it's going. In: ESRC UK Centre for Evidence Based Policy and Practice London.

Sorell, T. (2013). *Scientism: Philosophy and the infatuation with science*. Hoboken, NJ: Taylor and Francis.

Timmermans, S., & Berg, M. (2003). *The gold standard: The challenge of evidence-based medicine and standardization in health care*. Philadelphia, PA: Temple University Press.

Tjeltveit, A. C. (1999). *Ethics and values in psychotherapy*. London: Routledge.

Watson, J. B., & Watson, R. R. (1928). *Psychological care of the infant and child*. New York, NY: Norton.

Wells, H. G. (2017). *The island of Dr Moreau*. Oxford: Oxford University Press.

Wittgenstein, L. (2001). *Tractatus logico-philosophicus* (2nd ed.). Milton Park: Routledge.

World Health Organization. (1992). *The ICD-10 classification of mental and behavioural disorders: Clinical descriptions and diagnostic guidelines*. Geneva: World Health Organization.

3 The emergence of evidence-based medicine and the return of the expert

The use of evidence in medicine has a long history. Many consider Hippocrates (appx 460-377 BC) to be the founder of medicine. Hippocrates linked the treatment of symptoms to biological functions and to the interaction between environment and organism (Kleisiaris, Sfakianakis, & Papathanasiou, 2014). What distinguishes evidence-based medicine from thentofore medical models is not that it is rooted in evidence, but what type of evidence which is considered valid. Like many other sciences, medicine was established as a science in the contemporary meaning of that word in the 19th century. However, medicine was not very effective, which is illustrated by practices like bloodletting (Claridge & Fabian, 2005). A historic milestone in the history of medicine is the Flexner report, published in 1910. The report described and evaluated medical educational institutions in the United States and Canada. It revealed low standards and led to extensive reforms in medical education. In its wake, the number of educational institutions was reduced considerably, and medical education was standardised. The training became more scientifically oriented, and medicine gradually became an esteemed profession providing a good income. This, in turn, affected recruitment to attract good candidates. Thus, the Flexner report led to far better conditions for medical science and practice (Duncan & Reese, 2012).

The *direct* use of scientific evidence in medical practice, which characterises evidence-based medicine, has developed over time. One of the earliest known attempts to evaluate and criticise medical quality resembling evidence-based medicine is dated to 1912. However, for most of the 20th century, medicine was expert-based. The doctors' training and clinical experience was assumed to make medicine effective. Quality controls primarily identified unique errors committed by individual doctors (Goldman, 2002). The first versions of evidence-based medicine had a very different medical ideal. They were characterised by a sceptic stance to the clinical expert and emphasised the direct clinical value of science.

DOI: 10.4324/9781003512141-3

Archie Cochrane

Many consider Archie Cochrane (1909–1988) the originator of evidence-based medicine. Cochrane's medical thinking emanated from some personal experiences. As a prisoner of war during the Second World War, Cochrane was given medical responsibility for approximately 20,000 prisoners of war. The sanitary conditions were miserable. Viruses and bacteria flourished in the prison camp. Even though he did not have access to advanced medical equipment, very few patients died (only four of whom three were shot). At a later stage during the war, Cochrane gained access to more advanced medical equipment. However, he identified lack of knowledge as a limiting factor to turn the equipment into efficient practice.

These experiences inspired Cochrane to formulate a programme. It is described in *Effectiveness and Efficiency*, published in 1972 (thus, several decades after the Second World War). The text contains both political visions and an ideal for medical practice. Cochrane's overarching aim was to make public health services accessible to the entire population. To realise this vision, he believed it was necessary to identify effective and efficient interventions (Cochrane, 1999).

Cochrane criticised the assumption that traditional medical training and clinical practice ensure high-quality medical practice. He argued that medical practice should be tested directly and empirically. As Cochrane had suspected, empirical analyses revealed that medical practices often did have little effect. Cochrane concluded that medical treatment should be based directly on results from randomised controlled trials. By then, randomised controlled trials had already been established as the gold standard by The Food and Drug Administration (FDA) in the United States in the 1960s (Duncan & Reese, 2012). According to Cochrane, randomised controlled trials do not have the biases of clinical expertise. In other words, he claimed that randomised controlled trials show whether an intervention is effective. Cochrane's template can be found in empirically validated treatments, which preceded evidence-based practice in psychology (presented in Chapter 4).

Randomised controlled trials

Randomised controlled trials is a key method in several sciences. The first randomised controlled trial was published in 1948 (Meldrum, 2000). However, the undergirding logic of randomised controlled trials was known long before the emergence of modern science. The logic of randomised controlled trials was explicated by the British philosopher John Stuart Mill (1806–1873). Mill called it the 'method of difference' (Mill, 1843). If there is only one variable separating two phenomena, all observed differences in the phenomena must be due to this single variable.

In a healthcare context, we can rewrite this logical principle into a methodological principle. If two groups are identical except for one variable, all identified differences in the groups are caused by this variable. Thus, if two groups of patients are identical and only one group receives treatment, differences in symptoms between the groups after treatment completion must be attributed to the treatment. In other words, randomised controlled trials make it possible to infer causally. In healthcare research, a typical research question is whether a particular treatment form (e.g., psychotherapeutic intervention) has a specific effect (e.g., reduction of symptoms). Randomised controlled trials are conducted by comparing an experimental group and a control group. Randomisation reduces the number of systematic differences between the groups (ideally to a minimum). In addition, there must be experimental control; the conditions must be identical for both groups.

Let's say someone wanted to test whether a drug has an antidepressant effect. If the experimental group has milder depressive symptoms than the control group at the start of the study, it is unclear whether the observed difference (presuming there is one) is due to the antidepressant drug. The difference could be caused by the differences present before the start of the study. Likewise, if the control group receives the medicine from an empathic healthcare professional, while the control group is not in contact with any healthcare personnel, it will weaken the ability to infer causally. It may be the empathy (and not the antidepressant medications) which reduces the depressive symptoms.

The belief that one is receiving treatment can have a curative effect in itself (i.e., the placebo effect). Sometimes, RCTs have a placebo group receiving a so-called placebo control. From the example of the antidepressant drug, a placebo control would compare a group receiving the drug with putative active ingredients, with a group receiving a pill without the putative active ingredients (e.g., a sugar pill). If everything else is equal, the differences in symptoms between the group receiving the active ingredients and the group receiving a placebo can be attributed to the active ingredients (Brown, 2012). In healthcare contexts, it is necessary to identify the best means to realise specific goals. However, the final test for any intervention is practice, typically for a specific patient. Scientific knowledge only has practical value to the extent that it contributes to improve clinical treatment. This has also been a growing realisation within evidence-based medicine (in some of the later revisions).

Evidence-based medicine

Cochrane's criticism of expert-based medicine led to a series of critical analyses. Wennberg and Gittelsohn (1973) showed that there was substantial variability in the access to and use of healthcare services. This also applied to adjacent geographical areas. Other analyses revealed variability with fatal outcomes. Patients with early-stage prostate cancer were eight times more likely to have their prostate removed depending on whether they lived in two different locations in the United States (Baton Rouge and Tuscaloosa). In some areas of the United States, there was also a 33 times greater probability of receiving a treatment for breast cancer that was not the most well-documented one. Such random differences led to a demand for standardisation in healthcare services (Timmermans & Berg, 2003).

A group of researchers at the McMaster University (in Canada) were central to the development of evidence-based medicine. During the 1970s and 1980s, some researchers gave courses that focused on understanding the research findings based on epidemiology. Epidemiology maps factors related to health in a population. Typically, standardised quantitative measures logically equivalent to randomised controlled trials are used. Another topic was how to stay up to date given the large production of scientific knowledge. This topic has been very relevant during the past 50 years in which the research volume has increased drastically (Zimermann, 2013). In early stages, the group referred to the new approach to clinical practice as 'problem-based.' The choice of the term reflects the 'pragmatic spirit' in both evidence-based medicine and in evidence-based practice (miscellaneous) (Solesbury, 2001). Later, the group wrote several textbooks that introduce readers to the most central features of evidence-based medicine. One major publication is *Users' Guides to the Medical Literature* (Guyatt, Rennie, Meade, & Cook, 2014). Another is *Evidence-Based Medicine: How to Practice and Teach It* (Straus, Glasziou, Richardson, & Haynes, 2011). These books reflect that the training of students and professionals was one of the most important rationales for developing evidence-based medicine.

The term 'evidence-based medicine' itself was used in more and less formal settings during the 1980s, such as in seminars and at conferences. After first launching the term 'scientific medicine' (Sur & Dahm, 2011), Gordon Guyatt (1991) used the term 'evidence-based medicine' in a paper in 1991. However, it was not until 1992 – 20 years after Cochrane's publication of *Efficiency and Effectiveness* – that evidence-based medicine was formulated as a principle. A working group described evidence-based medicine as follows:

> A new paradigm for medical practice is emerging. Evidence-based medicine de-emphasizes intuition, unsystematic clinical experience, and pathophysiologic rationale as sufficient grounds for clinical decision making and stresses the examination of evidence from clinical research.
>
> (The Evidence-Based Medicine Working Group, 1992, p. 2420)

The working group was criticised for choosing the term 'paradigm.' Kuhnian paradigm shifts suggest radical changes. Paradigms are incommensurable.

This entails that the actors in different paradigms have problems in communicating. Taken literally, it would entail that the research carried out before evidence-based medicine has little or no relevance for evidence-based medicine (Goldenberg, 2006). The originators, and other key figures, de-escalated the rhetoric in more recent revisions. By the same token, the first version of evidence-based medicine do represent a shift from the expert-centred medicine that dominated prior to Cochrane and evidence-based medicine.

Revisions of evidence-based medicine

This first version of evidence-based medicine largely echoes Cochrane. Clinical practice is improved through the direct use of research. Randomised controlled trials are preferred as they contain unequivocal causal inferences. This model, however, was criticised for neglecting a number of issues related to translation (from scientific research to clinical practice) (Timmermans & Berg, 2003). Consequently, evidence-based medicine was expanded and redefined as:

> [...] the conscientious, explicit, and judicious use of current best evidence in making decisions about the care of individual patients.
> (Sackett, Rosenberg, Gray, Haynes, & Richardson, 1996, p. 312)

In this definition, some of the most central challenges of translating science to practice are addressed. First, it highlights that the clinical expert makes an assessment in the clinical consultation. Second, the patient is incorporated. It thus recognises that different patients with the same disease may have different (medical) needs. In addition, justice was included in the understanding of the best clinical practice. However, the two components 'clinical expertise' and 'patient' were embroidered in a text published a year later by David Sackett (1934–2015) (the first author of the text quoted above):

> Without clinical expertise, practice risks becoming tyrannized by external evidence, for even excellent external evidence may be inapplicable to or inappropriate for an individual patient [...] but [clinical expertise is] especially [important] in more effective and efficient diagnosis and in the more thoughtful identification and compassionate use of individual patients' predicaments, rights, and preferences in making clinical decisions about their care.
> (Sackett, 1997, pp. 3–4)

This led to a new tripartite model. This model consists of 'best external evidence,' 'clinical expertise,' and 'patient preferences.' The three components, moreover, are considered equally important in making good clinical decisions.

To specify what is meant by best evidence, different evidence hierarchies have been created ranking various research methods. At the top of this hierarchy of evidence, we usually find randomised controlled trials and compilations of several randomised controlled trials (e.g., systematic reviews, meta-analyses, mega-analyses). Typically, at the bottom is expert opinion. Since the revision incorporates clinical expertise as one of the three parts, the term '*external* evidence' has been chosen to denote *scientific* findings. In other words, there is a difference between expert opinion as external evidence and the utilisation of clinical expertise when treating an individual patient in the clinic. This differentiation arguably improved evidence-based medicine.

However, the evidence hierarchy in evidence-based medicine has been subject to revisions. In the *User's Guides to the Medical Literature*, Guyatt et al. (2014) describe a hierarchy of evidence where 'N-of-1' clinical trials are at the top. This is followed by randomised controlled trials, observational studies, basic research (laboratory experiments, animal experiments, and human physiology), and clinical expertise. In 'N-of-1' clinical trials, neither the patient nor the physician knows whether the patient is receiving assumed effective treatment or placebo. The reason why studies on single individuals is placed at the top is to reflect an ideal where treatment ideally is individualised. It is believed to be easier to achieve such information through direct individual testing of effect on the individual. However, this type of design has a very limited area of application. Nonetheless, it illustrates that evidence-based medicine is willing to reform (Guyatt, Rennie et al., 2014).

In addition, the authors describe an approach to evaluate research evidence called the GRADE approach. The GRADE classification indicates treatment effect (high, moderate, low, very low). The evidence hierarchy forms the starting point, but it is a final evaluation of the actual research that determines which GRADE classification. Randomised controlled trials are ranked as 'high.' However, if inferential biases are identified in a study, randomised controlled trials can be 'low' or even 'very low.' Furthermore, observational studies can end up in the classification 'moderate' and even 'high' if they are well-conducted. The differentiation between research design and actual research makes evidence-based medicine more sophisticated. A research design's potential is not as interesting as the quality of the actual research (Guyatt et al., 2014).

Clinical expertise

The second component of the revised model is clinical expertise. Clinical experts do not have research evidence to support all of their opinions or actions. Smith and Pell (2003) made a humoristic (if somewhat morbid) point of this fact in the paper entitled 'Parachute use to prevent death and major damage due to gravitational challenges.' In the paper, the researchers conducted a systematic literature review of the research investigating the relationship between parachute use and death:

> [...] parachutes have not been subjected to rigorous evaluation by using randomised controlled trials. Advocates of evidence-based medicine have criticised the adoption of interventions evaluated by using only observational data. We think that everyone might benefit if the most radical protagonists of evidence based medicine organised and participated in a double blind, randomised, placebo controlled, crossover trial of the parachute.
>
> (Smith & Pell, 2003, p. 1459)

The article shows that a medical practice based solely on scientific results is an unattainable ideal. We assume that causal relationships exist merely on the basis of everyday experience. Physicians also depend on other types of knowledge such as tacit knowledge (Polanyi, 2009; Thornton, 2006), procedural knowledge (Ryle, 1945), and bodily knowledge (Merleau-Ponty, 2004). Even one of the most sceptical thinkers in the history of philosophy, René Descartes, warned against radical scepticism thinking in everyday life. A radical sceptical attitude is not compatible with the uncertainty we have to accept in most practical contexts (Descartes, 2017).

Patient preferences and values

The last component of the revised version is patient's preferences and values. For a long time, medicine was paternalistic (Dworkin, 2013). In paternalistic healthcare practices, the expert decides on behalf of the patient. However, empirical research suggested that the clinical experts often make poor choices. In addition, educational levels rose in the end of the 20th century, improving patients' science literacy. In addition, information relating to the health profession became more available than before. The inclusion of patients in the decision-making processes is sometimes referred to as user involvement. User involvement is often regarded as a principal patient right. In that sense, the status of scientific evidence is subordinate to involving users in the decision-making process, which is in end in and by itself. In some cases, various treatment alternatives' effects are comparable. Yet, the risks or side effects may differ. Thus, the patient's preferences and values are central to decide the best treatment alternative (Llewellyn-Thomas, 2009). Decision-making tools have been developed to help inform the patient about various treatment options. The purpose of the decision-making tools is precisely to involve the patient in clinical decision-making (Elwyn et al., 2006; Elwyn et al., 2012) Patient preferences were also intended to be part of evidence-based practice in psychology. However, as we shall see, this is not realised in the current version of evidence-based practice in psychology.

The integrative clinical expert

In time, a new problem relating to the tripartite model was identified. The main rationale for expanding evidence-based medicine into a tripartite model was to make it more credible for clinical practice. What the tripartite model lacks, however, is an integrative body. If evidence-based medicine consists of the best external evidence, clinical expertise and the patient's preferences and values, the question remains: who will integrate them? Haynes, Devereaux and Guyatt's (2002) answer to this question was the clinical expert. Their revision of evidence-based medicine places the clinical expert at the centre stage. The three components (to be integrated) are revised to the best research evidence, the clinical circumstances and the patient's preferences and actions.

The article by Haynes et al. (2002) was published exactly 30 years after Cochrane's criticism of paternalistic medicine. At first glance, it may seem as if there is a full circle back to pre-Cochranian medicine. However, that is not the case. Although the clinical expert is the integrating body in the model by Haynes et al. (2002), it is nevertheless a model stating the importance of research evidence and a methodological hierarchy. In addition, it embodies patient's preferences and rights. Thus, it is a far more scientifically disciplined medical expert who must be responsive to individual variations within a patient group.

Conclusion

Medicine has changed drastically over the last 200 years. Evidence-based medicine constitutes one of its most important changes. In an unofficial award in the British Medical Journal, evidence-based medicine was voted the 8th most important medical innovation since 1840. However, evidence-based medicine has not only been important within medicine. It became a paradigmatic model for service delivery across sectors – even outside the healthcare sector. This has given rise to the characteristic 'evidence-based everything' (Fowler, 1997). Some examples of evidence-based practices are nursing (Ingersoll, 2000), policy-making (Solesbury, 2001), and law (Rachlinski, 2011). Even evidence-based alternative medicine exists (Borgerson, 2005).

The authors of evidence-based medicine were able to identify some genuine problems in medical practice. They have also succeeded in being self-critical and revising the model in the light of criticism. The important question is how to use the evidence-based medicine to inspire regulative principles in related practices such as psychotherapy. A key point is that a regulative principle is based on the nature of the practice. Then one must consider whether medicine has similar enough basic prerequisites that one should import a model from medicine to psychotherapy.

References

Borgerson, K. (2005). Evidence-based alternative medicine? *Perspectives in Biology and Medicine*, *48*(4), 502–515. https://doi.org/10.1353/pbm.2005.0084

Brown, W. A. (2012). *The Placebo effect in clinical practice*. Oxford University Press.

Claridge, J. A., & Fabian, T. C. (2005). History and development of evidence-based medicine. *World Journal of Surgery*, *29*(5), 547–553. https://doi.org/10.1007/s00268-005-7910-1

Cochrane, A. L. (1999). *Effectiveness and efficiency: Random reflections on health services*. London: Royal Society of Medicine Press.

Descartes, R. (2017). Principles of philosophy. Retrieved from http://www.earlymoderntexts.com/assets/pdfs/descartes1644part1.pdf

Duncan, B. L., & Reese, R. J. (2012). Empirically supported treatments, evidence-based treatments, and evidence-based practice. In G. Stricker, T. A. Wildiger, & A. B. Weiner (Eds.), *Handbook of psychology* (2nd ed., Vol. 8: Clinical psychology, pp. 489–514). Hoboken, NJ: Wiley.

Dworkin, G. (2013). Defining paternalism. In C. Coons & M. Weber (Eds.), *Paternalism: theory and practice* (pp. 25–38). Cambridge: Cambridge University Press.

Elwyn, G., Connor, A., Stacey, D., Volk, R., Edwards, A., Coulter, A., … Whelan, T. (2006). Developing a quality criteria framework for patient decision aids: online international Delphi consensus process. *British Medical Journal*, *333*(7565), 417. https://doi.org/10.1136/bmj.38926.629329.AE

Elwyn, G., Frosch, D., Thomson, R., Joseph-Williams, N., Lloyd, A., Kinnersley, P., … Barry, M. (2012). Shared decision making: A model for clinical practice. *Journal of General Internal Medicine*, *27*(10), 1361–1367. https://doi.org/10.1007/s11606-012-2077-6

Fowler, P. B. S. (1997). Evidence-based everything. *Journal of Evaluation in Clinical Practice*, *3*(3), 239–243. https://doi.org/10.1046/j.1365-2753.1997.00010.x

Goldenberg, M. J. (2006). On evidence and evidence-based medicine: Lessons from the philosophy of science. *Social Science and Medicine*, *62*(11), 2621–2632. https://doi.org/10.1016/j.socscimed.2005.11.031

Goldman, L. (2002). Alvan Feinstein: A tribute to quality and caring. *The American Journal of Medicine*, *112*(6), 502–503. https://doi.org/10.1016/S0002-9343(02)01039-2

Guyatt, G. (1991). Evidence-based medicine. *American College of Physicians Club Journal*, *114*(2), 16. https://doi.org/10.7326/ACPJC-1991-114-2-A16

Guyatt, G., Rennie, D., Meade, M. O., & Cook, D. J. (2014). *Users' guides to the medical literature: A manual for evidence-based clinical practice*. New York, NY: McGraw-Hill.

Haynes, B., Devereaux, P. J., & Guyatt, G. (2002). Clinical expertise in the era of evidence-based medicine and patient choice. *BMJ*, *136*, 383–386. https://doi.org/10.1111/j.1423-0410.2002.tb05339.x

Ingersoll, G. L. (2000). Evidence-based nursing: What it is and what it isn't. *Nursing Outlook*, *48*(4), 151–152. https://doi.org/10.1067/mno.2000.107690

Kleisiaris, C. F., Sfakianakis, C., & Papathanasiou, I. V. (2014). Health care practices in ancient Greece: The Hippocratic ideal. *Journal of Medical Ethics and History of Medicine*, *7*, 6–6. Retrieved from https://www.ncbi.nlm.nih.gov/pubmed/25512827; https://www.ncbi.nlm.nih.gov/pmc/articles/PMC4263393/

Llewellyn-Thomas, H. A. (2009). Values clarification. In A. Edwards & G. Elwyn (Eds.), *Shared decision-making in health care: Achieving evidence-based patient choice* (pp. 123–133). Oxford: Oxford University Press.

Meldrum, M. L. (2000). A brief history of the randomized controlled trial: From oranges and lemons to the gold standard. *Hematology/Oncology Clinics of North America*, *14*(4), 745–760, vii.

Merleau-Ponty, M. (2004). *The world of perception*. London: Routledge.

Polanyi, M. (2009). *The tacit dimension*. Chicago, IL: University of Chicago Press.

Rachlinski, J. J. (2011). Evidence-based law. *Cornell Law Review*, *96*(4), 901–923. Retrieved from http://scholarship.law.cornell.edu/clr/vol96/iss4/27

Ryle, G. (1945). Knowing that and knowing how. *Proceedings of the Aristotelian Society*, *46*, 1–16. Retrieved from http://www.informationphilosopher.com/solutions/philosophers/ryle/Ryle_KnowHow.pdf

Sackett, D. L. (1997). Evidence-based medicine. *Seminars in Perinatology*, *21*(1), 3–5. https://doi.org/10.1016/S0146-0005(97)80013-4

Sackett, D. L., Rosenberg, W. M. C., Gray, J. A. M., Haynes, R. B., & Richardson, W. S. (1996). Evidence based medicine: What it is and what it isn't. *British Medical Journal*, *312*(7023), 71–72. https://doi.org/10.1136/bmj.312.7023.71

Smith, G. C. S., & Pell, J. P. (2003). Parachute use to prevent death and major trauma related to gravitational challenge: Systematic review of randomised controlled trials. *British Medical Journal*, *327*, 1459–1461. https://doi.org/10.1136/bmj.327.7429.1459

Solesbury, W. (2001). Evidence based policy: Whence it came and where it's going. In *ESRC UK centre for evidence based policy and practice* London.

Straus, S. E., Glasziou, P., Richardson, W. S., & Haynes, R. B. (2011). *Evidence-based medicine: How to practice and teach it* (4th ed.). Edinburgh: Churchill Livingstone/Elsevier.

Sur, R. L., & Dahm, P. (2011). History of evidence-based medicine. *Indian Journal of Urology*, *27*(4), 487–489. https://doi.org/10.4103/0970-1591.91438

The Evidence-Based Medicine Working Group. (1992). Evidence-based medicine: A new approach to teaching the practice of medicine. *JAMA*, *268*(17), 2420–2425. https://doi.org/10.1001/jama.1992.03490170092032

Thornton, T. (2006). Tacit knowledge as the unifying factor in evidence based medicine and clinical judgement. *Philosophy, Ethics, and Humanities in Medicine*, *1*(2), 1–10. https://doi.org/10.1186/1747-5341-1-2

Timmermans, S., & Berg, M. (2003). *The gold standard: The challenge of evidence-based medicine and standardization in health care*. Philadelphia, PA: Temple University Press.

Wennberg, J., & Gittelsohn, A. (1973). Small area variations in health care delivery. *Science*, *182*(4117), 1102–1108. Retrieved from http://www.jstor.org/stable/1737008

Zimermann, A. L. (2013). Evidence-based medicine: A short history of a modern medical movement. *American Medical Association Journal of Ethics*, *15*(1), 71–76. https://doi.org/10.1001/virtualmentor.2013.15.1.mhst1-1301

Mill, John Stuart. 1843. *A System of Logic*. Vol. 1. London: Harrison and Co., Printers.

4 Evidence-based practice in psychology

Basing practice on evidence was not a new ideal in medicine and it is not a new ideal in psychotherapy either. Freud was inspired by natural sciences. Both Darwin's theory of evolution and Helmholtz's principle of energy conservation laid some of the foundation for his theory. An important reason why Freud built his theory on theories from the natural sciences was to legitimise psychoanalysis (Mitchell & Black, 1995).

Lightner Witmer created one of the world's first psychotherapy clinic (in the contemporary sense of the word) (Dreher, 2000). Like Freud, he appealed to science to advance clinical psychology (Witmer, 1996). Witmer is actually referred to in the policy statement for evidence-based practice in psychology (American Psychological Association, 2006). Witmer's ideals are also reflected in the Boulder model, which have influenced the training of psychotherapists to this day. At the Boulder conference (in the United States), the education of clinical psychologists was discussed. In the resulting Boulder model, training in clinical psychology consisted of a scientific and practical component. This means that candidates can do both research and clinical work after the completion of their studies (Baker & Benjamin, 2000).

However, both Freud's and Witmer's thinking exemplifies the fact that values permeate psychotherapy. According to Rieff, Freud struggled to balance scientific neutrality and humanistic reflexivity:

> An irrepressible moral earnestness colors his attitude of scrupulous scientific neutrality [...] [but]he could not avoid drawing morals from his diagnoses and influencing attitudes by his interpretations.
>
> (Rieff, 1961, p. 3)

Rieff claimed that an ethical purpose made it imperative for Freud to (try to) be strictly scientific. The purpose is to create a better life for the patients. Others have argued that Freud's thinking is an ethical theory in and by itself. Harcourt (2013) argued that Freud's psychoanalysis (and the psychodynamic tradition) has a natural place in a canon of normative

DOI: 10.4324/9781003512141-4

ethical theories. According to Harcourt, then, psychoanalysis is an ethical theory on a par with virtue ethics or utilitarianism. Despite Witmer's (1996) empirical focus, he described psychological ailments and disorders as 'moral problems' and 'moral disorders.' These terms reflect a particular conceptualisation of mental illness. Coining something a 'moral problem' entails claiming that certain behaviours are not desirable or acceptable. At least implicitly, it reflects standards for good and bad behaviour. To coin something a moral problem is not only to describe the world, but also to evaluate it. Such normative elements are also present in later psychotherapy therapists such as Carl Rogers (1902–1987), Rollo May (1909–1994), and Albert Ellis (1913–2007) (Ellis, 1962; May, 1983; Rogers, 1980, 1989) and in more modern approaches. In fact, as we shall see in Chapter 5, it is constitutive of psychotherapy as a practice.

Psychotherapy, science, and practice

In its beginning, clinical psychology was dominated by psychoanalytical and psychodynamic approaches. Some have described the dominance as total and that these traditions were enclosed and somewhat arrogant (Woolfolk, 2015). When behavioural and humanistic-existential approaches emerged and gained popularity, they challenged the psychoanalytic hegemony (Lambert, 2013). Lambert (2013) has linked the increasing concern with empirical evidence to the emergence of cognitive-behavioural therapy and the third edition of the DSM manual (DSM-III). Lambert (2013) argued that cognitive-behavioural therapy is a scientifically based therapy. In addition, the increasing specificity of the DSM-III made it significantly easier to test the effect of various treatment forms (Lambert, 2013). Westen, Novotny, and Thompson-Brenner (2004), who endorse scientifically based practice, have parodied the standard narrative of the history of psychotherapy and the transition from the 'old regime' to the 'new age':

> Once upon a time, in the Dark Ages, psychotherapists practiced however they liked, without any scientific data guiding them. Then a group of courageous warriors, whom we shall call the Knights of the Contingency Table, embarked upon a campaign of careful scientific testing of therapies under controlled conditions. Along the way, the Knights had to overcome many obstacles. Among the most formidable were the wealthy Drug Lords who dwelled in Mercky moats filled with Lilly pads. Equally treacherous were the fire-breathing clinician-dragons, who roared, without any basis in data, that their ways of practicing psychotherapy were better. After many years of tireless efforts, the Knights came upon a set of empirically supported therapies

> that made people better. They began to develop practice guidelines so that patients would receive the best possible treatments for their specific problems. And in the end, Science would prevail, and there would be calm (or at least less negative affect) in the land.
>
> (p. 631)

The parody stands as a reminder of a typical historical irony. Protest movements may end up having some of the features they arose to counteract. Robert Woolfolk is a cognitive behavioural therapist who, like the authors of the cited parody, argues that psychotherapy should be based on empirical research. Woolfolk (2015) has argued that the arrogance cognitive behavioural therapists found in psychoanalysis and psychodynamic therapy has become typical of adherents of cognitive-behavioural therapy too.

On the other hand, people in both the psychodynamic and humanistic/existential camps have expressed concern about the climate within the respective schools. Yalom and Lieberman (1971) investigated the effect of encounter groups and found that a significant proportion of clients experienced exacerbated symptoms. It illustrates the importance of scientific investigations. Although psychoanalytic or psychodynamic thinking was empirically tested as early as 1924 (Lambert, 2013), psychotherapists have not typically based their practices on research evidence such as randomised controlled trials.

Beutler (2000) argued that psychotherapy typically has been regulated through expert committees. Eysenck (1952) conducted one of the first meta-analyses investigating the effect of psychotherapy. He concluded that psychotherapy is ineffective and that psychoanalysis exacerbate symptoms. However, subsequent meta-analyses, using more robust data, have concluded that psychotherapy is an effective treatment form (Lambert, 2013). Lambert (2013) summarised the results as follows: ‘The effects of therapy are superior to no-treatment and placebo control conditions, and therapies appear to have equivalent effects when compared to each other across a variety of disorders’ (p. 5). While the conclusion is somewhat crude, these research results justify the use of psychotherapeutic treatment on a more general basis.

One question is whether psychotherapy has an effect. Another question, however, is *what* makes psychotherapy effective. A third discussion is *which methods* we should use to study psychological phenomena and which epistemological traditions the different methods are based on. A fourth question is the *relationship* between *scientific findings* and *clinical practice*; what parts of psychotherapy are addressed in scientific research. More or less explicitly, evidence-based practice in psychology answers all these questions.

Empirically validated treatments

Like evidence-based medicine (via Cochrane), evidence-based practice in psychology developed from an ideal according to which scientific findings should inform practice directly. But whereas evidence-based medicine follows from a critique of medicine, evidence-based practice in psychology arose from a confrontation with medicine (i.e., psychiatry). In the early 1990s, the American Psychiatric Association published guidelines for the treatment of various illnesses. The guidelines were based on expert opinions (Duncan & Reese, 2012). The clinical fractions in the American Psychological Association responded to make sure that psychotherapy (qua 'talking cure') could persist. The clinical division of the American Psychological Association therefore put together a working group:

> […] this task force was constituted to consider methods for educating clinical psychologists, third party payors, and the public about effective psychotherapies. Lacking the enormous promotional budgets and sales staff of pharmaceutical companies, clinical psychologists labor at a disadvantage to disseminate important findings about innovations in psychological procedures. Despite the great strides in the development and validation of effective treatments, it is not clear that the benefit of our approaches is widely appreciated, even by other clinical psychologists.
>
> (Chambless et al., 1993)

The working group established what was first launched as *empirically validated treatments* (Chambless et al., 1993; Chambless & Hollon, 1998). *Empirically validated treatments* have since been revised to *empirically supported treatments (Chambless, 1999; Chambless & Hollon, 1998; Chambless & Ollendick, 2001)* and again to *research-supported psychological treatments* (D. American Psychological Association, 2016).

The quotation shows that empirically validated treatments were first and foremost a strategic manoeuvre. Nonetheless, many psychologists welcomed the initiative. Robyn Dawes (1936–2010) argued that psychology had developed in a direction in which evidence gained an increasingly less prominent role in the three decades before empirically validated treatments emerged (Dawes, 1994). In the book entitled *House of Cards: Psychology and Psychotherapy Built on Myth*, he describes the situation as follows:

> […] there are big problems. *The question is whether the services rendered by professional psychiatrists and psychologists provide solutions to those problems* […] There is *some* scientific knowledge about some mental disorders and types of distress and how to alleviate them. When psychiatrists and psychologists base their practice on this knowledge, they

> generally perform a valuable service to their clients. All too often, however, mental health practitioners base their practice on what they believe to be an "intuitive understanding" of their clients' problems, an understanding they have supposedly gained "from experience." But when they practice on this intuitive basis, they perform at best as well as minimally trained people [...] and at worst as licensed, expensive (if inadvertent) frauds.
>
> (Dawes, 1994, pp. 8–9)

The working group intended to identify treatment methods for informing relevant actors and institutions. They had to establish criteria that made it possible to distinguish between well-informed and poorly informed (presumably good and poor) treatments. It is also worth noting that the quote claims that psychotherapists did not know the empirical research. Thus, it was a goal to ensure that psychotherapists became more empirically oriented and well-informed in their clinical work.

Empirically validated treatments consist of a list of treatment forms that have been tested empirically. Here, a treatment form means a psychotherapy school such as cognitive behavioural therapy, psychodynamic therapy, or existential therapy. Treatment forms are included in the list based on research that uses two different methodologies. The first is randomised controlled trials. The second is 'single case studies.' 'Single case studies' share the undergirding logic of randomised controlled trials but is a repeated measure design. (The same group is tested before and after and intervention. Before corresponds to the control group. After corresponds to the experimental group in a randomised controlled trial.) Depending on how many and what types of studies support the hypothesis that a treatment form is effective, it can be classified as a well-established treatment form or probably efficacious. The final product is a list of treatment forms that are effective for given psychiatric diseases.

The main rationale for revising empirically validated forms of treatment to empirically supported treatment was to avoid the denotations of the term 'validate.' It gives the impression that one can validate a treatment form once and for all. However, we cannot establish empirical claims once and for all, especially in sciences with complex objects of inquiry. Moreover, a complete overview of different treatment forms' effect is utopian due to the amount of research required. An estimation indicated that if there were 250 different schools of psychotherapy and 150 different types of psychiatric disorders, it would require 47 billion (47,000,000,000) studies to examine all the combinations of disorders and psychotherapy schools (Lambert, 2013). In fact, the estimate number of psychotherapy schools and psychiatric disorders is probably low in this example. In the transition from empirically validated forms of treatments to empirically supported forms of treatments, the inclusion criteria for the two levels ('well-established treatments' and 'probably efficacious treatments') were also modified. The latest revision, research-supported psychological treatments, is an internet site where clinicians and patients can consult and quickly get an overview of which psychotherapy schools have research support based on the two methods 'randomised controlled trials' and 'single case studies.' The criteria for being considered as a form of treatment with research support have not changed from empirically supported treatments.

Criticism of empirically validated treatments

Empirically validated treatments were criticised extensively (Bohart, O'Hara, & Leitner, 1998; Henry, 1998; Levant, 2004; Westen et al., 2004). Empirical psychotherapy research has been one source of criticism. This research shows that specific techniques associated with the various psychotherapy schools explain a modest proportion of the variance in psychotherapy's effect (Lambert & Barley, 2002). Exposure to an object (e.g., spiders) for which one has developed phobia is an example of a specific technique (often used in cognitive-behavioural therapy). However, other factors, transcending the various psychotherapy schools, can explain most of the therapy-related variance for outcomes in psychotherapy. These factors are coined common factors. Some examples of common factors are therapeutic alliance (e.g., affective bond, degree of agreement on process, and goals), empathy, and congruence (Norcross, 2011).

A study by Lambert and Barley (2002) showed that specific techniques only explain 15% of the variance in outcome (against common factors 30%, placebo/expectation 15% and extra-therapeutic factors 40%). In another study by Norcross and Lambert (2011), which included unexplained variance, the authors showed that the treatment method explain 8 % of the variance in outcome. In this study, 'patient factors' explained 30%, the therapeutic relationship explained 12%, the individual therapist explained 7%, and 'other factors' explained 3% of the variance (Norcross and Lambert, 2011). On this basis, critics argued that it is inappropriate to formulate a principle merely comparing psychotherapy schools.

Others have criticised the presupposition that standardisation is the key to good psychotherapy practice. First, empirically validated forms of treatments are based on single diagnoses. This does not reflect clinical practice in which patients are often comorbid (Aragona, 2009). Thus, it makes little sense to have a regulatory principle based on single diagnoses. Second, the clinical value of these treatment forms depends on the clinicians' ability to reproduce the clinicians in the empirical research (Westen et al., 2004). The latter criticism reflects the complexity in psychotherapy practice. We can contrast it with empirical research on psychopharmaceutical treatments. When testing a pill, there is less relevant variation from an experiment to clinical practice. However, in the case of psychotherapy (which typically lasts several weeks, months, or years), several factors will affect the treatment. Although there are manuals that describe treatments in detail, it is unlikely that manual-based psychotherapy will be performed identically or even similarly from one therapy series to another. Thus, critics claim that the high extent of standardisation does not fit clinical practice.

Some have criticised the conceptualisation of psychotherapy in empirically validated treatments. They argue that psychotherapy is understood as a 'pill' (Stiles & Shapiro, 1989). Of course, this also has methodological implications. When examining whether a pill is effective, randomised controlled trials can be highly relevant. However, psychotherapy practices are complex. Thus, RCTs (and their logical equivalents) are unable to describe all relevant facets of psychotherapy. Critics have argued that we need several different research designs to address relevant complexity.

Others have argued that psychotherapy is too dynamic to operate by a formalised criterion. As new forms of psychotherapy receive empirical support, it will be very difficult to keep such a list up to date and to disseminate it properly. In addition, it does not lead to (much needed) methodological innovation. Some psychotherapy researchers have also argued that empirically validated treatments reduce the number of forms of psychotherapy being offered. These critics argue that too little is known to exclude traditions with a long history in academia and in psychotherapy practice (Comer & Kendall, 2013; Lambert, 2013).

However, one text was particularly important for empirically validated treatments to be replaced by evidence-based practice in psychology. In the text *Science, scientism and professional responsibility*, Peterson (2004) discussed the relationship between science and practice. He claimed that scientific studies have limited relevance in complex practices like psychotherapy. Peterson (2004) contends that psychotherapy should be science-based, but that the translational inflexibility of empirically supported treatments is ill-founded. Ronald Levant (2004) praised the text for its description of the relationship between science and practice. Levant later became the first author of the American Psychological Association's policy statement for evidence-based practice in psychology. In other words, the background for introducing evidence-based practice in psychology was *to avoid the scientism in empirically supported treatments*. There were also empirical reasons related to parts of the above criticism, which led to the introduction of evidence-based practice in psychology:

> Suppose the profession had lists of empirically validated treatments for all *Diagnostic and Statistical Manual of Mental Disorders* Axis I diagnoses (which we are actually quite far from having). Practitioners would then have treatments for only a small minority of the patients

> who need our services, namely those who meet the diagnostic criteria used in studies that validated these treatments. To adequately serve this minority of patients, the average practitioner would have to spend many, many hours, perhaps years, in training to learn these treatments. And, in the end, these treatments would account for only 15% of the variance in therapy outcomes in these patients. One can readily see why many practitioners and even a noteworthy number of clinical educators are not able to uncritically embrace the empirically validated treatments movement.
>
> (Levant, 2004, p. 222)

To sum up, the scientific, methodological, empirical, and practical arguments against empirically validated treatments were overwhelming. Thus, it was abandoned in favour of a more comprehensive ideal.

Evidence-based practice in psychology

The American Psychological Association launched the policy statement for evidence-based practice in psychology in 2005. Early in the policy statement, reference is made to evidence-based medicine (Levant, 2005). Evidence-based practice in psychology, moreover, is an expansion of empirically validated treatments. Where empirically validated treatments entail basing practice directly on science, evidence-based practice in psychology (similar to the later revisions of evidence-based medicine) was intended to be tripartite. (In Chapter 7, however, we will see that evidence-based practice in psychology is not, in fact, a tripartite principle.)

The three components are 'best available research,' 'clinical expertise,' and 'patient characteristics, culture and preferences.' A key concept in the definition is 'integration.' For a practice to be evidence-based, these three components must be integrated. An important question is how we are to understand the prioritisation between the three components. Sometimes the evidence, the clinical expertise, and the patient's preferences will harmonise. Other times, however, they will conflict. In these situations, a crucial question is which element should carry most weight. There are no clear guidelines for how to solve such issues. However, the policy statement is coined evidence-based, and not expert-based or patient-based. The very name of the policy statement indicates its emphasis. According to Norcross, Hogan, and Koocher (2008), research evidence has precedence in evidence-based practice in psychology. However, the structure of the policy-statement begs the question: why should a three-partite principle where best available research is *one of the three* components be called *evidence-based practice* in psychology? If the aim was to integrate three components, it might be appropriate to find a new name that includes the entire content of the model, rather than merely one of its components.

Best available research evidence

The definition of best available research evidence (in evidence-based practice in psychology) is not clear-cut. This is somewhat remarkable. The policy statement centres around the concept of evidence. On the one hand, it includes different methods/designs. The methods/designs mentioned are:

- Clinical observation
- Qualitative research
- Systematic case studies
- Experimental single case studies
- Public health studies and ethnographic research
- Process-outcome research
- Studies of interventions delivered / performed in naturalistic settings
- Randomised controlled trials
- Meta-analyses

The policy statement acknowledges that these research methods/designs have complementary strengths and weaknesses. However, the range of methods/designs is by no means exhaustive of the methods/designs relevant to psychotherapy. The selection is somewhat random, and the degree of specificity is variable.

While it recognises the value of different types of research, the policy statement includes a methodological hierarchy: 'Clinical observation (including individual case studies) and basic psychological science are valuable sources of innovations and hypotheses' (American Psychological Association, 2006, p. 274). Clinical observations can generate hypotheses that should be tested using other methods. Thus, clinical observation is not considered a credible source of knowledge in and by itself.

The policy statement is explicitly hierarchical regarding research on so-called specific interventions. The policy statement contains two evaluation criteria for research on specific interventions. One is effectiveness and the other is efficiency. These parameters reflect Cochrane's medical ideals. They are also central in evidence-based medicine. Effect refers to the scientific evidence in support of an intervention. Efficiency includes the practical implementation of particular interventions. It includes practical feasibility (e.g., clinical competence) and cost-effectiveness. In the evaluation of specific interventions, the evidence hierarchy from evidence-based medicine is at work:

> Types of research evidence with regard to intervention research in ascending order as to their contribution to conclusions about efficacy include "clinical opinion, observation, and consensus among recognized experts representing the range of use in the field" (Criterion 2.1);

> "systematized clinical observation" (Criterion 2.2); and "sophisticated empirical methodologies, including quasi experiments and randomized controlled experiments or their logical equivalents Among sophisticated empirical methodologies, "randomized controlled experiments represent a more stringent way to evaluate treatment efficacy because they are the most effective way to rule out threats to internal validity in a single experiment."
>
> (Criterion 2.3; American Psychological Association, 2002, p. 1054)

It is worth dwelling on the understanding of best evidence. Evidence-based practice in psychology is explicitly based on the template of evidence-based medicine. One of evidence-based medicine's most central features is the evidence hierarchy. The description of the various methodologies indicates that randomised controlled trials are deemed superior (like in evidence-based medicine). It maintains that randomised controlled trials can verify scientific propositions, indicating their special status. In psychotherapy, moreover, the distinction between a specific intervention and facilitating factors is unclear. An example could be a psychotherapist who actively tries to establish a good relationship with the patient. Would that be a specific intervention or a facilitating factor? This conceptual unclarity fundamentally blurs when the narrower evidence hierarchy applies (privileging randomised controlled trials) and not.

The ambiguity of the term 'specific intervention' impedes a critical debate about evidence-based practice in psychology. In response to accusations of a narrow conception of science, advocates of evidence-based practice in psychology can reply that several methodologies are included in the policy statement. At the same time, (based on) randomised controlled trials and 'evidence-based' are sometimes used synonymously. In the end, it is the role of the various methodologies in clinical practice that is decisive.

Clinical expertise

As we have seen, the first evidence-based medicine models emerged as a response to paternalistic ideals. The same can be said for empirically validated treatments. It sought to remedy that clinical practice was expert-based and that practitioners lacked empirical knowledge (Chambless et al., 1993). Reintroducing clinical expertise means acknowledging that the clinical expertise is instrumental to clinical practice. At the same time, the understanding of clinical expertise in evidence-based practice has been characterised as poorly developed (Norcross et al., 2008). We will revert to this topic in Chapters 7 and 8.

A clinical expert has extensive knowledge and practical skills. It is often presumed that there is a positive correlation between experience and expertise. In addition, there are several clinical factors that science does not address. Science consists of theories entailing abstraction. The theories generally require some adaptation for clinical practice. When translating scientific findings into clinical practice, the clinical expert plays a crucial role. This was recognised by some of the pioneers in evidence-based medicine (describing scientific findings as a potential tyrant in clinical practice).

There has been a tension between theoretical models and clinical practice since the pioneering days of psychotherapy. Freud's ideal of an abstinent therapist is a good example. According to Freud, psychoanalysts should be impersonal. Freud uses the metaphor of a mirror when describing the analyst; the analyst should merely reflect the patient (Freud, 1912). However, personal accounts and letters show that Freud himself was in fact personal in psychotherapy. He probably developed clinical skills owing to that being personal could be expedient (despite being inconsistent with his own theoretical model) (Lohser & Newton, 1996). Recent empirical research also indicates that different forms of personal involvement may impact psychotherapy outcomes positively (Berg, Antonsen, & Binder, 2016; Norcross, 2011; Wampold, 2011).

Woolfolk (2015) has argued that practitioners with an unsophisticated understanding of science has become a growing problem in psychotherapy. Woolfolk was a student under the pioneers in cognitive-behavioural therapy. He argued that these pioneers always adapted their interventions to the practical context. However, the one-sided focus on scientific evidence has led subsequent generations to utilise science directly. According to Woolfolk, this weakens the quality of clinical work because scientific theories must always be adapted, requiring an active clinical expert (Woolfolk, 2015).

The clinical expert must be able to translate the scientific knowledge to different clinical situations. At the same time, clinical expertise exceeds propositional knowledge. A clinical expert has different forms of knowledge that differs from scientific knowledge (e.g., tacit knowledge, contextual knowledge, procedural knowledge) (Fulford, 2013; Polanyi, 2009; Ryle, 1945; Wittgenstein, 1958, 1969). Clinical expertise for a psychotherapist is characterised not least by ethical knowledge, in the sense of knowing what the right action in a particular context is (Berg & Slaattelid, 2017; Pellegrino & Thomasma, 1993; Waring, 2016). As we will see in Chapter 8, however, this is neglected in evidence-based practice in psychology.

The patient's culture, characteristics, and preferences

The last component is the patient's characteristics, culture, and preferences. The patient's cultural background emphasises the importance of a particular patient characteristic – generally a very significant one. However, it is important to note that many other specific patient characteristics can also be of great importance in psychotherapy. Some examples are gender, age, or socioeconomic status. Moreover, there is a fundamental difference between the patient's characteristics and culture on the one hand, and patient preferences on the other. The patient's characteristics and culture say something about how the patient is like. One can inform the treatment and culture by using empirical research on how culture and specific characteristics affect treatment. However, patients' preferences refer to what individual patient wants and must therefore always be examined as individual preferences. Thus, it is the patient's preferences (which could be shaped by characteristics and culture) that is the crucial element in this component. The main purpose is that the patient has a say in the treatment.

Patient preferences are linked to the ethical concept autonomy. Autonomy literally means 'self-legislation.' It is a key ethical principle in today's thinking about healthcare (Beauchamp & Childress, 2009). Although there are important differences between preferences and autonomy, it is impossible to have patient autonomy without including patient preferences. Therefore, the patient preferences play an important ethical role in psychotherapy. The patient's preferences are also linked to user rights. User rights include a right to influence all levels of the health services offered, including the knowledge base for the health services. User participation represents a very strong contrast to the expert-based models that previously dominated healthcare practices. User involvement serves as a reminder that healthcare services primarily exist to help patients with their unique challenges.

Conclusion

Evidence-based practice in psychology emerged in a confrontation with medicine. The American Psychological Association created a model built on evidence-based medicine. However, while evidence-based medicine has been the subject to several revisions, evidence-based practice in psychology has not been revised since its adoption. An important reason for this may be that evidence-based practice in psychology has been subject to surprisingly few critical analyses. However, when we consider the importance of evidence-based practice in psychology, this is puzzling. Evidence-based practice in psychology aims to raise the quality of psychotherapy practice. Consequently, it is crucial to carry out critical analyses of how evidence-based practice in psychology functions. In the following chapters, evidence-based practice in psychology will be criticised on different grounds. The ultimate aim is to formulate some basic pillars for an improved principle that is not based on strategic concerns, but on the nature of psychotherapy. The first thing we must do is to try to characterise the nature of psychotherapy (the topic of Chapter 5).

References

American Psychological Association. (2006). Policy statement on evidence-based practice in psychology. *American Psychologist*, *61*(4), 271–285. http://doi.org/10.1037/0003-066X.61.4.271

American Psychological Association (2016). Research-supported psychological treatments. Retrieved from https://www.div12.org/psychological-treatments/

Aragona, M. (2009). The role of comorbidity in the crisis of the current psychiatric classification system. *Philosophy, Psychiatry, & Psychology*, *16*(1), 1–11. http://doi.org/10.1353/ppp.0.0211

Baker, D. B., & Benjamin, L. T., Jr. (2000). The affirmation of the scientist-practitioner: A look back at Boulder. *American Psychologist*, *55*(2), 241–247. http://doi.org/10.1037/0003-066X.55.2.241

Beauchamp, T. L., & Childress, J. F. (2009). *Principles of biomedical ethics* (6th ed.). Oxford: Oxford University Press.

Berg, H., Antonsen, P., & Binder, P.-E. (2016). Sediments and vistas in the relational matrix of the unfolding "I": A qualitative study of therapists' experiences with self-disclosure in psychotherapy. *Journal of Psychotherapy Integration*, *26*(3), 248–258. http://doi.org/10.1037/a0040051

Berg, H., & Slaattelid, R. (2017). Facts and values in psychotherapy: A critique of the empirical reduction of psychotherapy within evidence-based practice. *Journal of Evaluation in Clinical Practice*, *23*(5), 1075–1080. http://doi.org/10.1111/jep.12739

Beutler, L. E. (2000). David and Goliath: When empirical and clinical standards of practice meet. *American Psychologist*, *55*(9), 997–1007. http://doi.org/10.1037/0003-066X.55.9.997

Chambless, D. L. (1999). Empirically validated treatments – What now? *Applied & Preventive Psychology*, *8*(4), 281–284. http://doi.org/10.1016/S0962-1849(05)80043-5

Chambless, D. L., Babich, K., Crits-Christoph P., Frank E., Gilson M., Montgomery R. (1993). Task force on promotion and dissemination of psychological procedures. Retrieved from http://www.div12.org/sites/default/files/InitialReportOfTheChamblessTaskForce.pdf

Chambless, D. L., & Hollon, S. D. (1998). Defining empirically supported therapies. *Journal of Consulting and Clinical Psychology*, *66*(1), 7–18. http://doi.org/10.1037/0022-006X.66.1.7

Chambless, D. L., & Ollendick, T. H. (2001). Empirically supported psychological interventions: controversies and evidence. *Annual Review of Psychology*, *52*, 685–716. http://doi.org/10.1146/annurev.psych.52.1.685

Comer, J. S., & Kendall, P. C. (2013). Methodology, design and evaluation in psychotherapy research. In M. J. Lambert (Ed.), *Bergin and Garfield's handbook of psychotherapy and behaviour change* (6th ed., pp. 21–48). Hoboken, NJ: John Wiley & Sons.

Dawes, R. M. (1994). *House of cards: Psychology and psychotherapy built on myth*. New York, NY: Free Press.

Dreher, A. U. (2000). *Foundations for conceptual research in psychoanalysis*. London: Karnac Books.

Duncan, B. L., & Reese, R. J. (2012). Empirically supported treatments, evidence-based treatments, and evidence-based practice. In G. Stricker, T. A. Wildiger, & A. B. Weiner (Eds.), *Handbook of psychology* (2nd ed., Vol. 8: Clinical psychology, pp. 489–514). Hoboken, NJ: Wiley.

Ellis, A. (1962). *Reason and emotion in psychotherapy*. Secaucus, NJ: Lyle Stuart.

Eysenck, H. J. (1952). The effects of psychotherapy: An evaluation. *Journal of Consulting Psychology*, *16*(5), 319–324. http://doi.org/10.1037/h0063633

Freud, S. (1912). Recommendations for physicians on the psychoanalytic method of treatment. In P. Rieff (Ed.), *Therapy and technique* (pp. 117–126). New York, NY: Collier Books.

Fulford, K. W. M. (2013). Values-based practice: Fulford's dangerous idea. *Journal of Evaluation in Clinical Practice*, *19*(3), 537–546. http://doi.org/10.1111/jep.12054

Harcourt, E. (2013). The place of psychoanalysis in the history of ethics. *Journal of Moral Philosophy*, *10*(4), 598–618. http://doi.org/10.1163/17455243-4681030

Lambert, M. J. (2013). Introduction and historical overview. In M. J. Lambert (Ed.), *Bergin and Garfield's handbook of psychotherapy and behaviour change* (6th ed., pp. 3–20). Hoboken, NJ: John Wiley & Sons.

Lambert, M. J., & Barley, D. E. (2002). Psychotherapy relationships that work: Evidence-based responsiveness. In J. C. Norcross (Ed.), *Psychotherapy relationships that work* (pp. 17–32). New York, NY: Oxford University Press.

Levant, R. F. (2004). The empirically validated treatments movement: A practitioner/educator perspective. *Clinical Psychology: Science and Practice*, *11*(2), 219–224. http://doi.org/10.1093/clipsy.bph075

Levant, R. F. (2005). *Report of the 2005 Presidential Task Force on evidence-based practice*. Retrieved from https://www.apa.org/practice/resources/evidence/evidence-based-report.pdf

Lohser, B. M., & Newton, P. M. (1996). *Unorthodox Freud: The view from the couch*. New York, NY: Guilford Press.

May, R. (1983). *The discovery of being: Writings in existential psychology*. New York, NY: Norton & Company.

Mitchell, S. A., & Black, M. J. (1995). *Freud and beyond: A history of modern psychoanalytic thought*. New York, NY: Basic Books.

Norcross, J. C. (2011). *Psychotherapy relationships that work: Evidence-based responsiveness* (2nd ed.). New York, NY: Oxford University Press.

Norcross, J. C., Hogan, T. P., & Koocher, G. P. (2008). *Clinician's guide to evidence based practices: Mental health and the addictions*. New York, NY: Oxford University Press.

Norcross, J. C., & Lambert, M. J. (2011). Evidence-based therapy relationships. In J. C. Norcross (Ed.), *Psychotherapy relationships that work: Evidence-based responsiveness* (2nd ed., pp. 3–24). New York, NY: Oxford University Press.

Pellegrino, E. D., & Thomasma, D. C. (1993). *The virtues in medical practice*. New York, NY: Oxford University Press.

Peterson, D. R. (2004). Science, scientism, and professional responsibility. *Clinical Psychology: Science and Practice*, *11*(2), 196–210. http://doi.org/10.1093/clipsy.bph072

Polanyi, M. (2009). *The tacit dimension*. Chicago, IL: University of Chicago Press.

Rieff, P. (1961). *Freud: The mind of a moralist*. New York, NY: Anchor Books.

Rogers, C. (1980). *A way of being*. Boston, MA: Houghton Mifflin Company.

Rogers, C. (1989). *On becoming a person: A therapist's view of psychotherapy*. New York, NY: Mariner Books.

Ryle, G. (1945). Knowing that and knowing how. *Proceedings of the Aristotelian Society*, *46*, 1–16. Retrieved from http://www.informationphilosopher.com/solutions/philosophers/ryle/Ryle_KnowHow.pdf

Stiles, W. B., & Shapiro, D. A. (1989). Abuse of the drug metaphor in psychotherapy process-outcome research. *Clinical Psychology Review*, *9*(4), 521–543. http://doi.org/10.1016/0272-7358(89)90007-X

Wampold, B. (2011). *Qualities and actions of effective therapists*. Retrieved from https://www.apa.org/education/ce/effective-therapists.pdf

Waring, D. R. (2016). *The healing virtues*. Oxford: Oxford University Press.

Westen, D., Novotny, C. M., & Thompson-Brenner, H. (2004). The empirical status of empirically supported psychotherapies: Assumptions, findings, and reporting in controlled clinical trials. *The Psychological Bulletin*, *130*(4), 631–663. http://doi.org/10.1037/0033-2909.130.4.631

Witmer, L. (1996). Clinical psychology: Reprint of Witmer's 1907 article. *American Psychologist*, *51*(3), 248–251. http://doi.org/10.1037/0003-066X.51.3.248

Wittgenstein, L. (1958). *Philosophical investigations* (2nd ed.). Oxford: Blackwell.

Wittgenstein, L. (1969). *On Certainty*. New York, NY: Harper & Row.

Woolfolk, R. L. (2015). *The value of psychotherapy: The talking cure in an age of clinical science*. New York, NY: The Guilford Press.

Yalom, I. D., & Lieberman, M. A. (1971). A study of encounter group causalities. *Archives of General Psychiatry*, *25*(1), 16–30. http://doi.org/10.1001/archpsyc.1971.01750130018002

5 Facts and values in psychotherapy

Psychotherapy has been based on empirical data since its pioneering times. Yet, it is only of late that effect studies have become the state of the art. The first randomised controlled psychology experiments were carried out at the end of the 19th century (Peirce & Jastrow, 1884). Nonetheless, randomised controlled experiments were not common in psychology until around the 1970s (Lambert, 2013). As already noted, research carried out over several decades indicated that psychotherapy works. We have also touched upon the discussions regarding what makes psychotherapy work (Chambless & Crits-Christoph, 2006; Wampold, 2001, 2011, 2015). Some researchers argue that the specific techniques (related to the various psychotherapy schools) make psychotherapy work. A good example is exposure (to feared objects) in cognitive-behavioural therapy (Chambless and Crits-Christoph, 2006). Others claim that effective therapy is characterised by some common factors existing across different psychotherapy schools (e.g., the therapeutic alliance, empathy, congruence) (Wampold, 2001).

Wampold (2001) coined this discussion 'the great psychotherapy debate.' Which therapeutic actions are associated with given outcomes is indeed an important question. More high-quality empirical research is needed to illuminate it. By the same token, there is a question that is even 'greater' for the understanding of psychotherapy. It is the question of what kind of practice psychotherapy is or what 'being effective' even means. This question – arguably, the most central aspect of psychotherapy – is not thematised in evidence-based practice in psychology (nor in empirical validated treatments). In this chapter, we will take a closer look at which role values and ethics play in psychotherapy.

Facts and values

One of the main topics in philosophy is the relation between facts and values. Ideal types present the world in distinct categories. However, the phenomena represented in ideal types might not be as distinct. We can think of facts and values as ideal types. Facts describe state of affairs.

DOI: 10.4324/9781003512141-5

They say something about how the world is like (e.g., 'The cat is grey'). However, facts do not say anything about how the world should be like. Values, on the other hand, are evaluations. Value statements may be aesthetic (e.g., 'The house is beautiful'), moral (e.g., 'That was mean'), or practical (e.g., 'The tap is not working'). We may attribute value to both objects, humans, actions, or conduct of life. Moreover, values are related to normative points of view. A normative point of view says something about how something *ought* to be, without necessarily giving a description of how something is (e.g., 'everybody should be kind'). In short, descriptive statements describe and normative statements evaluate.

There is also a dividing line between moral and ethics. Moral normally refers to widespread understandings of bad and good and/or right and wrong. One example may be how mental illness was and is perceived in society at large. Traditionally there has been stigma associated with mental illness (Byrne, 2001). Note that morality does not tell us anything about goodness or rightness per se. Morality simply describes perceptions of what is good or right.

Ethics, on the other hand, provides analyses of the good and bad and/or right and wrong. However, there are different branches of ethics. Descriptive ethics is empirical analyses of actual attitudes and values related to different questions. In other words, it is empirical analyses of morality. An example of descriptive ethics could be an empirical survey showing that there is less stigma associated with mental illness in 2020 as compared to 1960. Normative ethics consists of theories describing what characterises the good and bad and/or the right and wrong. Normative ethics is thus a level of analysis that does not (necessarily) include moral perceptions. We may for example argue that (it is right that) everybody is treated equally (normative ethics), even though all groups are not treated equally (morality).

Even though they are describing different levels of analysis, both morality, descriptive ethics and normative ethics can be related in intricate ways. It is for example likely that a certain era's moral code affects normative ethics. It is no coincident that the duty ethicist Immanuel Kant (1724–1804) lived in the Age of Enlightenment. This era emphasised the human potential for emancipation through critical thinking (Kant, 1997). Normative ethics also affects morality. That is to say, theories of 'goodness' and 'rightness' influence peoples' perception of good and bad and right and wrong. Kantian ideals of autonomy (normative ethics) influence the way contemporary societies think about patient rights.

The history of philosophy contains various theories addressing the relationship between facts and values. The philosopher David Hume (1711–1776) proposed an absolute division between facts and values. According to Hume, nobody (before him) had been able to make a clear division between 'is' and 'ought' statements. He claimed that descriptive statements derive from reasons and that normative statements stem from our emotions. When we evaluate, it is in other words an expression of emotion (Hume, 2009). Hume's absolute division between descriptive and normative statements was reintroduced in logical positivism. Like Hume, certain logical positivists claimed that the normative content of statements is 'meaningless' (Ayer, 1936, 1959). This conceptualisation of facts and values has influenced a *scientistic* conception of psychotherapy (Tjeltveit, 1999).

The German sociologist and philosopher Max Weber argued that science should be value neutral. However, the historical background for Weber's thinking is important. Some of Weber's predecessors claimed that there was a *single* correct answer in normative questions that could be revealed by empirical investigations. This means that they assumed that science could *determine* political questions. Science can help us identify good means, but it cannot identify good aims. Weber claimed that the question of 'goodness' and 'rightness' belongs to ethics and not science.

Douglas (2009) argued that the value free ideal was less influential after Weber passed away in 1920. Merton's (1910–2003) 'The normative structure of science' discusses the role of facts and values in science. In this text, Merton (1973) described the ethos of science through four scientific norms. The term 'ethos' refers to normative principles that form the basis for a certain activity (here science). The four norms in Merton's article (1973) are 'universalism,' 'organised scepticism,' 'communality,' and 'disinterestedness.' Even though 'disinterestedness' is related to value freedom, the two terms do not have identical meaning. It is possible to recognise that values constitute a part of science without actively seeking to promote certain values. This is the meaning of 'disinterestedness' (Merton, 1973). Moreover, Merton (1973) upheld that these fours norms thrive in democratic societies, as opposed to totalitarian societies. Consequently, Merton claimed that the governance of science and society is related (Douglas, 2009).

According to Douglas (2009), events in the wake of the Second World War corroborated the value-free ideal:

> [...] even as [some scholars] presented clear arguments for the importance of values in science, pressures to professionalize the young discipline of philosophy of science took hold. Arguments that scientists should only consider values internal to science were made. The idealized image of the isolated scientific community gained prominence [...] Although some criticisms of the value-free ideal have persisted, they have been ignored or marginalized by the philosophers of science. And the ideal has been influential among scientists [...].
>
> (p.65)

The value-free ideal is based on a certain relation between science and society. It is assumed that science and society are two distinct domains with little contact. In addition, there were also strategic concerns involved. If science is a specialised domain, this legitimises a group of specialists (i.e., philosophers of science) analysing science.

The French philosopher and social anthropologist Bruno Latour (1993) linked the separation of facts and values to modernity. Modernity sought to establish an absolute division between facts and values. On the one hand, there is science, nature, and facts. On the other hand, there is politics, society, and values. However, in an essay with the title 'We have never been modern', Latour (1993) claimed that modernity is based on an illusion. We have never been modern in the sense that these two dimensions never were separated. Science, nature, and facts have always been entangled with politics, science, and values. We may have good reasons to try isolate them to the extent possible under certain historical, social, and political conditions. However, this does not mean that the two dimensions ever become separate. When we investigate what makes psychotherapy effective, we want to test the proposition as objectively as possible. However, it is probably in the interest of the government (who might have funded the study) to identify more efficient health services. Even when it's carried out in an unbiased manner, psychotherapy research is political. Psychotherapy can be an important political instrument to ensure employment, rehabilitate prisoners, or in treating addictions. Psychotherapy also reflects certain moral and cultural values related to conduct of life (Tjeltveit, 1999, 2004). The connection between 'science, nature and facts' and 'politics and values' become visible when we use scientific studies to inform political decisions. The same holds true when political authorities want to make evidence-based policies (Latour, 1993).

The value-free ideal shapes the perception of reality, including practices like psychotherapy. However, the fact that science is mobilised to test propositions does not make psychotherapy value free. Science may inform decisions but can never determine what the 'good' decision is. When utilising scientific findings, one must take into consideration what is incorporated in a scientific study and what is not. The statements that are tested in psychotherapy research are value-laden; psychotherapy is pervaded by values. This has not been recognised in evidence-based practice in psychology (nor in empirically validated treatments).

Psychotherapy and professional ethics

Clinical psychology is tied to ethical frameworks and legal documents. These regulate psychologists and patients' rights and obligations. This type of ethical framework belongs to a branch of ethics called applied ethics (Beauchamp, 2003; Singer, 2011). Another related term is professional ethics. Professional ethics thematises ethical problems related to a particular professional practice like clinical psychology.

Applied ethics links ethics (typically normative ethics) to specific practical problems. One example is: 'When is it permissible to compromise confidentiality?' Another is: 'What kind of patients should be prioritised in healthcare?' Several different normative ethical theories can inform applied ethics. One example is the balancing of inviolable right (e.g., the right to privacy) with the best possible consequences (e.g., good health). This example balances duty ethics and utilitarianism in normative ethics. Balancing patient autonomy (irrespective of outcome) and empirically informed good outcomes (regardless of the patient's preferences) is another example.

As psychotherapy became increasingly popular after the Second World War, the American Psychological Association developed an ethical code. The ambition was to create an ethical code that could assist clinicians in integrating ethical problems into clinical practice. An empirical approach was preferred because it was more practically oriented than abstract (top-down) principles based on normative ethics. In addition, it was believed that clinicians would feel more akin to an ethical code based on the practice itself. However, early documents emphasised that the underlying philosophical perspective must be elucidated (Hobbs, 1948). We can suppose that this would lead us into normative ethics and, thus, that normative ethics is necessary to really understand the ethical codes properly.

Tjeltveit has identified three main problems relating to the traditional professional ethics. First, they often exclude patients and other relevant groups when they are created. Thus, important perspectives are probably excluded from ethical codes. Second, the focus of professional ethics has been too narrow to address the relevant ethical problems in psychotherapy. Professional ethics typically consist of 'codes' or regulatory ethical principles but that cannot say much about the purpose of psychotherapy. Third, ethical codes do not normally give reasons for *why* an ethical principle is important. It may (correctly) prohibit professionals from having intimate relations with their patients, yet without stating the reasons why this is right or good (Tjeltveit, 1999). These three factors contribute to a distorted ethical regulation of psychotherapy. In addition, it leads to an impoverished conception of psychotherapy.

Ethical principles

The American Psychological Association (American Psychological Association, 2017b) has created ethical principles to regulate clinical practice. Among these, there are five general ethical principles:

- Beneficence and non-maleficence
- Fidelity and responsibility
- Integrity
- Justice
- Respect for people's rights and dignity

These principles reflect Beauchamp and Childress' (2009) four principles of bioethics (1. Beneficence, 2. Non-maleficence, 3. Respect for autonomy, and 4. Justice). Bioethics is the ethics of the life sciences (particularly medicine). In the five principles set out by the American Psychological Association (2017), facts and values are to some degree integrated. 1. Beneficence and non-maleficence do comprise an ethical assessment of research practices. 2. Integrity is concerned with the ethical obligation to be truthful. Nonetheless, psychotherapy is still characterised by a lack of understanding of *how* important moral and ethics are (American Psychological Association, 2017b). This most certainly also applies to evidence-based practice in psychology.

What is psychotherapy?

Phenomenology may help clarify which type of activity psychotherapy is. Many phenomenologists describe a pre-scientific background constituting the conditions of possibility for science. To access this pre-scientific foundation, phenomenology describes that which appears and how it appears (Heidegger, 1962; Husserl, 1970). If we apply this to psychotherapy, the role that normative statements play in psychotherapy practice become evident. In psychotherapy, the patient's and the psychotherapist's statements are generally normative. Evaluations are often the basis for the description of the patient's condition (e.g., 'I sleep *badly*,' 'I am not doing *well*,' 'I have been more *anxious* this week'). It is also often the basis for the therapist's response (e.g., 'maybe sleep routines can help you sleep *better*,' 'what do you think could make you feel *better*?', 'that sounds rather *unpleasant*'). In addition, the normative dimension of psychotherapy is indicated from non-verbal actions such as a patient crying or having a restless body.

A vignette from a psychotherapy session may help illustrate the point. In the following case vignette, the patient is a war veteran receiving cognitive-behavioural therapy for post-traumatic stress disorder (PTSD):

Therapist *Jill, do you mind if I ask you a few questions about this thought that you noticed, "I should have had them wait and not had them go on?"*

Client *Sure.*

Therapist *Can you tell me what the protocol tells you to do in a situation in which a truck breaks down during a convoy?*

Client *You want to get the truck repaired as soon as possible, because the point of a convoy is to keep the trucks moving so that you aren't sitting ducks.*

Therapist *The truck that broke down was the lead truck that you were on. What is the protocol in that case?*

Client *The protocol says to wave the other trucks through and keep them moving so that you don't have multiple trucks just sitting there together more vulnerable.*

Therapist *Okay. That's helpful for me to understand. In light of the protocol you just described and the reasons for it, why do you think you should have had the second truck wait and not had them go on?*

Client *If I hadn't have waved them through and told them to carry on, this wouldn't have happened. It is my fault that they died. (Begins to cry)*

Therapist *(Pause) It is certainly sad that they died. (Pause) However, I want us to think through the idea that you should have had them wait and not had them go on, and consequently that it was your fault. (Pause) If you think back about what you knew at the time — not what you know now 5 years after the outcome — did you see anything that looked like a possible explosive device when you were scanning the road as the original lead truck?*

Client *No. Prior to the truck breaking down, there was nothing that we noticed. It was an area of Iraq that could be dangerous, but there hadn't been much insurgent activity in the days and weeks prior to it happening.*

Therapist *Okay. So, prior to the explosion, you hadn't seen anything suspicious.*

Client *No.*

Therapist *When the second truck took over as the lead truck, what was their responsibility and what was your responsibility at that point?*

Client *The next truck that Mike and my other friends were on essentially became the lead truck, and I was responsible for trying to get my truck moving again so that we weren't in danger.*

Therapist *Okay. In that scenario then, would it be Mike and the others' jobs to be scanning the environment ahead for potential dangers?*

Client *Yes, but I should have been able to see and warn them.*

Therapist *Before we determine that, how far ahead of you were Mike and the others when the explosion occurred?*

Client *Oh (pause), probably 200 yards?*

Therapist *200 yards—that's two football fields' worth of distance, right?*

Client *Right.*

Therapist *You'll have to educate me. Are there explosive devices that you wouldn't be able to detect 200 yards ahead?*

Client *Absolutely.*

Therapist *How about explosive devices that you might not see 10 yards ahead?*

Client *Sure. If they are really good, you wouldn't see them at all.*

Therapist *So, in light of the facts that you didn't see anything at the time when you waved them through at 200 yards behind and that they obviously didn't see anything 10 yards ahead before they hit the explosion, and that protocol would call for you preventing another danger of being sitting ducks, help me understand why you wouldn't have waved them through at that time? Again, based on what you knew at the time?*

Client *(Quietly) I hadn't thought about the fact that Mike and the others obviously didn't see the device at 10 yards, as you say, or they would have probably done something else. (Pause) Also, when you say that we were trying to prevent another danger at the time of being "sitting ducks," it makes me feel better about waving them through.*

Therapist *Can you describe the type of emotion you have when you say, "It makes me feel better?"*

Client *I guess I feel less guilty.*

Therapist *That makes sense to me. As we go back and more accurately see the reality of what was really going on at the time of this explosion, it is important to notice that it makes you feel better emotionally. (Pause) In fact, I was wondering if you had ever considered that, in this situation, you actually did exactly what you were supposed to do and that something worse could have happened had you chosen to make them wait?*

Client *No. I haven't thought about that.*

Therapist *Obviously this was an area that insurgents were active in if they were planting explosives. Is it possible that it could have gone down worse had you chosen not to follow protocol and send them through?*

Client *Hmmm. I hadn't thought about that either.*

Therapist *That's okay. Many people don't think through what could have happened if they had chosen an alternative course of action at the time or they assume that there would have only been positive outcomes if they had done something different. I call it "happily ever after" thinking — assuming that a different action would have resulted in a positive outcome. (Pause) When you think, "I did a good job following protocol in a stressful situation that may have prevented more harm from happening," how does that make you feel?*

Client *It definitely makes me feel less guilty.*

Therapist *I'm wondering if there is any pride that you might feel?*

Client *Hmmm…I don't know if I can go that far.*

Therapist *What do you mean?*

Client *It seems wrong to feel pride when my friends died.*

Therapist *Is it possible to feel both pride and sadness in this situation? (Pause) Do you think Mike would hold it against you for feeling pride, as well as sadness for his and others' losses?*

Client *Mike wouldn't hold it against me. In fact, he'd probably reassure me that I did a good job.*

Therapist *(Pause) That seems really important for you to remember. It may be helpful to remind yourself of what you have discovered today, because you have some habits in thinking about this event in a particular way. We are also going to be doing some practice assignments that will help to walk you through your thoughts about what happened during this event, help you to remember what you knew at the time, and remind you how different thoughts can result in different feelings about what happened.*

Client *I actually feel a bit better after this conversation.*

(American Psychological Association, 2017a).

Several aspects of the vignette are noteworthy. First, the therapist focuses on convincing the patient that she acted morally or ethically correct. To achieve this, the therapist points to the empirical facts. According to the therapist, a major part of the patient's problem is that she has distorted the facts and thus concluded erroneously. Second, the vignette contains several normative terms. The starting point is something the patient believes that she 'shouldn't' have done. In other words, it describes a moral or ethical obligation that the patient did not live up to. The patient's guilt is caused by the distance between the ideal action and the choice of action. The therapist seems to believe the guilt is unjustified and thus should be replaced by other, more adequate, emotions. The adequate emotions are grief or sadness, not guilt. Additionally, the therapist encourages the patient to feel pride for having acted in a good and/or right way in an extremely demanding situation. Towards the end of the vignette, the patient concludes that she is feeling better after the conversation. This is interpreted as a sign that the intervention was successful.

What is characteristic of the vignette is that the success criteria for the therapy is inseparably linked to certain normative standards. In this case, that the patient should think differently about the question of guilt. Given the importance of the memory, changing it will probably also change the patient's self-image (and, presumably, her life). However, this presupposes certain standards for what we consider to be good and right. More than anything, the vignette demonstrates that it is impossible to understand the interaction between the patient and the therapist without using normative concepts.

In the vignette, the therapist refers to a rule of action which increases the chances for good results in combat. Because the patient followed that rule of action, her action was good. However, we could have had different normative criteria to evaluate her actions. We could have argued that it is the result of the action that determines whether the action is good or bad (not the rule). According to such criteria, the patient's action could have been assessed as a bad action because it resulted in loss of life. To add to the complexity: even if they had assessed the action as bad, the therapeutic work could have developed in different ways. The therapist and the patient could have argued that bad actions are a part of being human and reduced (what they at the time were thinking of as damaging) perfectionism. However, they could also have focused on how to improve. Psychotherapy sometimes involves 'improvement' of various kinds (e.g., reduce violent conduct or harmful addictions). The understanding of 'goodness' and 'rightness' is decisive for the assessments and the conclusions. The normative ideals provide fine-meshed guidelines for therapeutic assessments and choices of action.

In addition, there are several other factors that influence the evaluation of the actions in the vignette. One is the question of loyalty. What kind of loyalty is most important for the patient? Is it the loyalty to fellow soldiers? Her next in kin? Her country? Or maybe humanity, in general? The conflict that the patient is part of will also influence our assessment of the above actions. Is it a justified conflict or a controversial conflict? These are just some factors influencing how we would evaluate the actions of the patient.

As psychotherapy is entrenched with normative questions, psychotherapists (and patients) have two options. Either the normative standards can work implicitly. Or one can try to explicate them. Surely, few if anyone would deem it acceptable to treat patients according to implicit normative standards. Thus, we should try to clarify the normative standards in the practice of psychotherapy.

Psychotherapy and normativity

Psychotherapy is based on a fundamental normative principle. This fundamental normative principle is that a life without (or with an altered relation to) mental illness or suffering is better than *status quo*. If psychotherapy does not aim to reduce (or change the relation to) mental illness or suffering, psychotherapy is a futile enterprise. The rationale for the activity is the prospect of a better life. How psychotherapy may contribute towards improvement is, however, far more ambiguous than this premise.

A main problem that evidence-based practice in psychology and empirically validated treatments face is the parameters used for evaluating psychotherapy. In evidence-based practice in psychology and empirically validated treatments, only scientific findings are considered relevant to evaluate psychotherapeutic interventions. However, science cannot answer normative questions directly. The physicist and philosopher of science Alvin Weinberg (1972) introduced the term 'trans-science' to describe scientific questions that cannot be answered by science alone. This is a type of question that is particularly relevant in social and health sciences which contain both facts and values. A comprehensive understanding of psychotherapy must include its aims.

Ethos in psychotherapy

The various schools of psychotherapy are founded on different ethoses. These ethoses are relatively distinct normative standards. They answer questions like 'what is a human-being?', 'what characterises a good development from childhood to adult life?', 'what is the nature and cause of mental illnesses?', 'what is the relation between an individual and other human beings?', 'what characterises the good life?', 'what is the relation between body and mind?', 'what is the relation between rationality and emotions?', to mention some (Berg and Slaattelid, 2017). Various psychotherapy schools emphasise some normative questions more than others. Yet, every psychotherapy school (and psychotherapy as such) is founded on an ethos (i.e., a set of normative standards). In other words, pure empirical evaluation criteria are insufficient to evaluate and understand psychotherapy.

It may be useful to illustrate this point using some examples. As we have seen, the American Psychological Association (2016) operates with five main approaches to psychotherapy. The five main approaches are behavioural therapy, cognitive therapy, psychoanalytic/psychodynamic therapy, humanistic-existential therapy, and eclectic or integrative therapy (American Psychological Association, 2016). Eclectic or integrative therapy are approaches which combine elements from different traditions and/or are based on empirical findings (e.g., the common factors) (Fernandez-Alvarez, Consoli, & Gomez, 2016). To illustrate this point, we shall take a closer look at the ethos of three main psychotherapy schools: cognitive-behavioural therapy, relational psychodynamic therapy, and existential therapy. In addition, we will analyse integrative psychotherapy.

It is important to emphasise that there is a great variation within these schools; neither cognitive-behavioural therapy, psychodynamic therapy, or existential therapy are uniform traditions. There are also revised versions that emerged from these schools (e.g., metacognitive therapy). In addition, there are hybrids of different schools of psychotherapy. An example is mindfulness-based cognitive-behavioural therapy (combining mindfulness and cognitive-behavioural therapy). Consequently, none of the following descriptions will neither be indisputable nor exhaustive. However, the main point of the descriptions is to illustrate that psychotherapy schools have ethoses.

The ethos of cognitive-behavioural therapy

Cognitive-behavioural therapy combines behavioural psychology and cognitive psychology. Behavioural psychology typically describes how associations between 'various stimuli' and 'stimuli and responses' affect behaviour. Cognitive psychology has a wider scope including topics like sensation, perception, thinking, memory, and behaviour. Aron T. Beck (the founder of cognitive-behavioural therapy), however, had his clinical training in psychoanalysis. Beck examined some of the psychoanalytical assumptions empirically but did not find any empirical support for them. From Beck's further work, cognitive-behavioural therapy was created (Beck Institute for Cognitive Behavior Therapy, 2019). Critics have claimed that empirically validated treatments (as well as evidence-based practice in psychology) favour cognitive-behavioural therapy (Bohart, O'Hara, & Leitner, 1998). Moreover, cognitive-behavioural therapy is the most frequently cited psychotherapy school on the list of empirically validated treatments (or research-supported psychological treatments) (American Psychological Association, 2016).

However, both cognitive-behavioural therapy and its forerunners are indebted to ethics. The influence of ethics was acknowledged by several central scholars in the history of (what has later become) cognitive-behavioural therapy. Some examples are Paul Dubois (1829–1905), Hans Eysenck (1916–1997), Donald Meichenbaum (Robertson, 2010), and Albert Ellis (1913–2007). The latter, who founded a forerunner to cognitive-behavioural therapy called rational emotive therapy, wrote the following:

> Many of the principles incorporated in the theory of rational-emotive psychotherapy are not new; some of them, in fact, were originally stated several thousand years ago, especially by the Greek and Roman stoic philosophers (such as Epictetus and Marcus Aurelius). [...] What is probably new is the application to psychotherapy of viewpoints (such as these) that were first propounded in radically different contexts.
>
> (Ellis, 1962, p. 35)

Aron T. Beck acknowledged that stoic principles undergird cognitive-behavioural therapy. In *Cognitive Therapy and Emotional Disorders*, he wrote:

> These assumptions converge on a relatively new approach to emotional disorders. Nevertheless, the philosophical underpinnings of this approach go back thousands of years, certainly to the time of the Stoics, who considered man's conceptions (or misconceptions) of events rather than the events themselves as the key to his emotional upsets.
>
> (A. T. Beck, 1976, p. 3)

The stoic quotes belong to ethics. An important distinction in stoic ethics runs between what you can influence and what you cannot. A key to good living is the ability to accept what you cannot change. As we presumably have greater control of our perception of the world (as opposed to the world itself), it will be easier to change our perception of the world (rather than the world itself). Consequently, the difference between appearance and occurrence is decisive (Epictetus, 2014). A quote from Bennet-Levy et al. (2004) may illustrate the affinity:

> Cognitive theory suggests that psychological disorders do not arise from events per se (e.g., a traumatic incident or the loss of a job or relationship). Problems arise from the meanings individuals give to events, filtered through the framework of core beliefs and assumptions which they have already developed through life experience.
>
> (p. 4)

In other words, a central tenet in cognitive-behavioural therapy is that mental illness is caused by dysfunctional thinking. Cognitive-behavioural therapy focuses on automatic thoughts and core beliefs. Automatic thoughts are thoughts that appear without voluntary control. Core beliefs are often deeper assumptions which structure the individual's interpretations (e.g., 'I am worthless') (Bennett-Levy et al., 2004). Judith S. Beck (2011) writes: 'When people learn to evaluate their thinking in a more realistic and adaptive way, they experience improvement in their emotional state and in their behaviour' (p. 3). In cognitive-behavioural therapy, one of the main goals is to minimise the emotions that: 'interferes with a patient's capacity to think clearly, solve problems, act effectively, or gain satisfaction' (J. S. Beck, 2011, p. 158). Cognitive-behavioural therapy has similarities with virtue ethics (which stoic ethics exemplifies). Virtue ethics defines goodness in terms of certain character traits (i.e., virtues). According to the 'ethos' of cognitive-behavioural therapy, central character traits to live a good life are rationality and autonomy. This harmonises with the demands put on individuals in modern Western societies. Critics have argued that cognitive-behavioural therapy is symptomatic of a neo-liberal ideology where the individuals are held responsible for his or her own life. This is problematic when individual's problems are caused by social conditions (and not the individuals themselves) (Madsen, 2015).

A premise in cognitive-behavioural therapy is that our thoughts should be tested systematically and empirically to determine their rationality. George Kelly (1905–1967) used the metaphor of a scientist to describe human beings. Generally speaking, human beings test and revise their believes (Winter, 2013). In behavioural experiments, patients test 'catastrophic thinking.' Catastrophic thinking is a negatively laden prediction linked to a certain action or situation (e.g., 'I always embarrass myself'). The empirical test investigates the prediction (Bennet-Levy et al., 2004). In empirical testing, specificity is key. One example of catastrophic thinking could be 'If I enter the bus, others will ridicule me.' To test this presumption, the patient is requested to enter the bus to see if in fact the other passengers will start smiling scornfully or laughing. The empirical tests make the patient able to conduct realistic evaluations without the distortions of mental illness.

Cognitive-behavioural therapy typically focuses on symptoms rather than aetiology. Robins and Block (1989), however, described cognitive-behavioural therapy as a stress-diathesis model. Stress-diathesis models emphasise the interaction between biological factors and (in particular early) life events, as well as later life stressors. The combination is deemed decisive for whether an individual will develop mental illness (Bennet-Levy et al., 2004). Thus, vulnerable individuals may develop mental illness due to smaller stressors. More robust individuals develop mental illnesses due to significant stressors. Moreover, in cognitive-behavioural therapy, mental illness is understood similarly to somatic disorders. Mental illness should be minimised and ideally removed. Mental illness is considered to deviate from a normative normal condition which will only be re-established when the pathological symptoms disappear.

The therapist (and other persons) is considered 'helpers' or 'facilitators.' This is in line with Bandura's social learning theory, which emphasises the importance of observational learning (Benjamin et al., 2011) In cognitive-behavioural therapy, other persons may function as models (Goldfried, Burckell, & Eubanks-Carter, 2003) The goal is to improve the patients' ability to help themselves by use of various techniques. One of the central therapeutic techniques is 'Socratic questioning.' The term refers to the Greek philosopher Socrates, who sought to unlock dormant potential in his interlocutors (Plato, 2010). Through cognitive-behavioural therapy, the patient ideally understands the nature of and solution to the illness (Clark & Egan, 2015). Even more important is the acknowledgement that the patient must choose to think or act differently. It requires discipline to endure unpleasant exposure, and it requires dedication to change one's mindset. The psychotherapist can explain why this is advisable, but it is ultimately the patient who must make the choice.

Cognitive-behavioural therapy typically ends when the patient has sub-clinical scores on standardised inventories. Inventories have been developed and tailored for cognitive-behavioural therapy such as 'Beck's depression inventory' and 'Beck's anxiety inventory,' which measure depression and anxiety symptoms, respectively (A. T. Beck, Epstein, Brown, & Steer, 1988a; A. T. Beck, Steer, & Carbin, 1988b). After the end of treatment, some patients get less intensive therapy for maintaining the low levels of symptoms.

The ethos of relational psychodynamic therapy

Psychodynamic therapy is an umbrella term for various traditions which have their historical origins in Freudian psychoanalysis. The basis for classical psychoanalysis is that human beings have two basic drives. These drives are sexual (i.e., libido) and aggressive (i.e., thanatos). Classical psychoanalysis describes the human psyche as an ongoing struggle and balancing of basic internal drives and external normative standards. In Freud's structural model, these instances are id (i.e., basic drives), ego (i.e., mediator), and superego (i.e., external normative standards). There are many potential conflicts in the balancing processes of the ego. Mental illness arises when the tension between the drives and the external standards is handled inadequately (Freud, 1961).

In relational psychodynamic therapy, it is assumed that the human psyche is relational. Stolorow and Atwood (1992) write:

> [W]e challenge a central myth that pervades contemporary Western culture and has insinuated itself into the foundational assumptions of psychoanalysis – The Myth of the Isolated Individual Mind. By bringing into focus the unconscious organizing power of this myth and proposing an alternative perspective emphasizing the intersubjective foundations of psychological life, we hope to contribute [...] to the advancement of psychoanalytic theory.
>
> (p. 7)

Stolorow and Atwood (1992) link the myth of the isolated human mind to Cartesian philosophy. Descartes distinguished between consciousness (in Latin, *res cogitans*) and matter (in Latin, *res extensa*). Due to Descartes' influence, there is a tendency to think of the human psyche as individual (particularly in Western countries) (Stolorow and Atwood, 1992). The individualisation is reflected in classical psychoanalysis' distinction between internal drives and external normative standards. However, in relational psychodynamic therapy our minds are inherently relational. We are not biological beings who adapt to social institutions. We are social beings who understand our biology through relational structures.

Like classical psychoanalysis, relational psychodynamic thinking describes the human psyche as layered. The human mind has a conscious part that we can access quite easily. In addition, it contains unconscious structures that are much harder to identify. Whereas the conscious part typically has a specific (albeit often relatively fluctuating) content, the unconscious part structures the very patterns in our thoughts, feelings, and actions. We can imagine a person (let's call her 'Anne') disappointed by the way a close friend reacts when 'Anne' experiences loss. 'Anne' may think that her friend does not like her anymore. Consequently, she decides to avoid the friend. This may reflect a characteristic way of interpreting incidents structured by the unconscious. 'Anne' could have reacted with anger and actively confronted the friend. 'Anne' may have thought that the friend did not live up to the expectations of a close friend, which in turn reflects a more self-assertive pattern. The examples illustrate that the unconscious structural level is of great importance to how we feel about ourselves and others.

The unconscious structures are shaped by the interactions with primary caregivers. Mental illness is primarily caused by various experiences which structure the unconscious level adversely. Examples can be lacking emotional 'attunement' for certain emotions (Stern, 1985), primary care givers' lacking recognition and confirmation of a child's self-worth (Brandchaft & Stolorow, 1994) or even more serious cases such as psychosis after sexual abuse (Davies & Frawley, 1991).

Naturally, it is difficult for patients themselves to identify the unconscious structures. Nonetheless, these structures must be identified to change them. In psychotherapy, the patient's unconscious structures are analysed and identified as they unfold in therapy (with the therapist). Through analyses, the therapist and the patient can come to gain an understanding of the unconscious structures. Because the unconscious structures are revealed in a specific therapist–patient-dyad, however, both personality structures influence what is being revealed. Consequently, it is also important for the therapist to understand his/her own contribution to the therapeutic interaction. The therapist's reactions are coined countertransference. Analysing the countertransference is pivotal to the analytic work (Hayes, Gelso, Goldberg, & Kivlighan, 2018; Maroda, 1991). It is important to discern which patterns that are particular to a therapist–patient-dyad and what reflects the patient more generally. In addition, the therapist's focus on his or her influence helps the patient think about him/herself as a relational being (i.e., in relation to others).

According to relational psychodynamic theory, mental illness occurs when the individual deviates from a natural (and good) development. A good development occurs when the caregiver balances several different needs. One example is the balance between security and independence. In attachment theory, the metaphor 'secure base' is used to describe the good caregiver. The child should be able to use 'the secure base' to regulate his/her feelings when exploring the world (Adshead, 2018). The contact with the primary caregiver is presumably decisive for emotional development. A child who does not get positive emotions reciprocated (for example by a depressed mother) may develop an inadequate emotional register which may lead to emotional problems (throughout life) (Lichtenberg, 2003). Another example is the balance between rationality and affect. In psychodynamic theory, emotions are not subordinate to the rational part of the human psyche in healthy individuals (this contrasts with cognitive-behavioural therapy). In the psychodynamic tradition, the transition from the affective characterising infants to the more rational and verbal adulthood is something of a trade-off. In these transitions, significant affective vitality is lost (Mitchell, 2000).

Within the psychodynamic tradition, mental illness is considered less binary than in cognitive-behavioural therapy. While mental illness should be reduced, it acknowledges that symptoms of mental illness are universal human features. However, in the psychodynamic tradition, the focus is less on descriptive diagnoses (which is more prominent in cognitive behavioural therapy) and more on aetiology (Lingiardi & Bornstein, 2017; McWilliams & Shedler, 2017). Through analysing the unconscious, psychotherapy enables patients to understand themselves. Insight makes new reactions, emotions, and actions possible (Pérez-Rojas et al., 2017). The intention is to facilitate an improvement in the patient's life. On the one side, this takes place through new experiences together with the therapist. On the other hand, it improves through understanding the relational patterns. Compared to cognitive-behavioural therapy, there is less instrumentalism in the psychodynamic tradition. A greater diversity of human interests is sought realised in psychotherapy. Thus, it does not always fit the standardisation requirements in evidence-based practice in psychology.

The ethos of existential therapy

While both cognitive-behavioural therapy and psychodynamic therapy arose as psychotherapeutic traditions, existential therapy emerged from the philosophical and literary tradition called existentialism. This tradition varies with a view to many questions. One recurrent question in existentialism, however, is the question of meaning. One of the things that separate human beings from other animals is that we do not simply live, we also ascribe meaning to events. This puts us in a unique position as we also may pose the question of the meaning of life – that is, of why we exist.

The French philosopher Albert Camus (1913–1960) used the Greek 'Myth of Sisyphus' to describe the human situation. Sisyphus is a character from Greek mythology who is condemned to push the same boulder up a mountain. When he gets to the top, the boulder rolls down and Sisyphus has to start the same process over again. This process is repeated eternally. According to Camus, the myth of Sisyphus is a metaphor of the human situation. The only way for Sisyphus to endure is to attribute meaning to his destiny. It is futile to *search for* the meaning of life; the meaning must, according to Camus, be created (Camus, 2002).

Existential philosophers often analyse the question of meaning through characters (who illustrate the attempt to answer this question through different life projects). One example is the philosopher Soren Kierkegaard (1813–1855) (Kierkegaard, 1987). The characters in his philosophy have different ultimate concerns. An ultimate concern is the deepest motivation for an individual's choice of action (Tillich, 1958). For some of these characters, it is to obtain hedonistic pleasure, for others relational devotion and for others again it is pure will to power. It is characteristic that Kierkegaard does not end up concluding plainly. Like life itself, uncertainty and ambiguity pervade the analysis. A central goal in existential therapy is to learn how to live with the uncertainty of life (Jacobsen, 2007).

In existential therapy, mental illness is primarily linked to loss of meaning. The modern industrialised world has solved many problems for parts of the population, particularly in Western countries. At the same time, there is an increasing instrumentalisation of human existence itself. This has led to an alienation described in Franz Kafka's novels. In the novels, the main character struggles with a fundamental confusion. The mood is not merely unpleasant (or unhomely, as many existentialists would say), it is difficult to identify what the actual problem is. This is symptomatic for existential thinking. Our problems do not exist in organised categories. Consequently, it may be necessary with a considerable amount of analytical work to establish a good understanding of the challenges of a concrete existing human being.

Existentialists' understanding of meaning is tied to our finitude. Martin Heidegger (1889–1976) describes the human (in his nomenclature *there-being*) situation as characterised by us interpreting and reinterpreting our history and future through the present. Human life is full of potential, also for re-interpreting the lives we have lived. The 'most certain possibility' is that one day life will end. This is why angst has a central role in existentialism. Whereas fear is directed towards specific objects or situations, angst is the intensely unpleasant experience that is (in contrast to fear) not linked to specific objects. Angst signals our finitude in a confronting and overwhelming manner (May, 1983). It forms, moreover, the basis for human responsibility and new ways to relate to our existence. In the existentialist literature, this is often referred to as authenticity. Heidegger argued that most aspects of human existence is cultural and social. Death, in contrast, is individual. And, thus, it signals our individuality. This also opens us up, phenomenologically speaking, to new ways of being. Thus, angst (despite being uncomfortable) and authenticity have therapeutic potential (Heidegger, 1962).

Whereas mental illness is conceptualised as something that should be removed or reduced in cognitive-behavioural therapy and psychodynamic therapy, existential thinking emphasises that suffering is integral to human life. In contrast to, for example, positive psychology (Seligman & Csikszentmihalyi, 2000), several philosophers in the existential tradition consider life itself to be a problem. Humans are 'thrown' into life with needs. At the same time, need satisfaction will not necessarily lead to contentment. The accountability of humans is also concerned with confronting life, as it *is* – also the inevitable unpleasant sides of living (Nietzsche, 2012).

Existential philosophers are concerned with human existence. In contrast, other theories attempt to describe human essences. According to Heidegger (1962), human beings share some fundamental structures. However, these structures must be understood in their unique and individual existence. All humans have a body, are part of a social community, learn a language from a linguistic community, and so on. Nonetheless, human beings must be understood in their unique existence. This point is relevant because it makes standardising far less relevant in psychotherapy. Humans are unique individual creatures with individual and unique needs. A person's anger, frustration, or grief are not manifest expressions for some universal latent emotions. They must be understood as they manifest individually (Guignon, 2006).

Because the distinction between the pathological and the normal is less clear-cut in existential therapy, there is no obvious ending point in therapy. Even though the existential tradition generally emphasises the grim aspects of existence, there are also existential philosophers who emphasise creativity and freedom. If human existence is not conditioned by an essence, this also means that humans are free to create their own meaning. The American philosopher Richard Rorty (1931–2007) (paraphrasing Nietzsche) expresses it as a move from 'how it was' to 'how I willed it' (Rorty, 1989). We do not need to look for the truth behind the manifest expressions as there is nothing to look for: the essence is the existence itself. One central goal in psychotherapy is to embrace the human opportunities, by confronting the conditions of life.

The ethos of psychotherapy integration

There are differences and similarities in the normative basis for the psychotherapy schools outlined above. The main point, however, is that *all* psychotherapy schools are founded on a normative basis (i.e., an ethos). To describe a psychotherapy school, this normative basis must be included.

One of the five main approaches identified by the American Psychological Association is integrative approaches to psychotherapy. Integrative approaches are often divided into four sub-approaches.

- The common factors approach is therapy based on the common factors (e.g., the therapeutic alliance, empathy, etc.).
- Assimilative integration takes a given psychotherapy school as its point of departure, while including elements from other schools. An example could be a relational psychodynamic therapist who treats a patient by exposure therapy (typically used in cognitive-behavioural therapy).
- Technical eclecticism means using techniques from various schools flexibly.
- Theoretical integration means creating new theoretical perspectives integrating elements from existing theoretical perspectives. An example of theoretical integration is mindfulness-based cognitive therapy.

(Stricker, 2010)

Although it may be harder to identify the ethos of integrative psychotherapy, it is nevertheless based on an ethos. This ethos cannot be outlined through empirical facts. As we have already seen, the two alternatives are to let it take effect implicitly or to explicate it.

However, the task of identifying values in psychotherapy is demanding. Tjeltveit (1999) claims that both explicit and implicit values shape psychotherapy. Certain values are expressed quite clearly through the schools of psychotherapy, but there are other values involved in psychotherapy as well. Tjeltveit (1999) writes: ‘values that are rarely examined, values perhaps subtly conveyed in the language, symbols, stories, and institutions of psychotherapy, values perhaps so widely or deeply held in a particular culture that they remain unnoticed’ (p.4). At the same time, we must strive to illuminate the values that form the basis of psychotherapy. While we will probably never be able to identify *all* the values or settle what it is ‘the correct’ values. We should nonetheless strive to have a truthful conceptualisation of psychotherapy as value laden. This is important both to the professional and the public understanding of psychotherapy.

Conclusion

One main problem in evidence-based practice in psychology and empirically validated treatments is the implicit conceptualisation of psychotherapy. Psychotherapy cannot be evaluated by scientific findings alone. Science may help to identify efficient means. However, it is unsuited to establish the aims of psychotherapy. There are different legitimate objectives in psychotherapy. To be able to discuss these, we must include normative concepts and ethical theory. The 'ethos' of psychotherapy, which describes the most central normative elements of psychotherapy, is at the heart of this discussion. This is a different way of thinking about psychotherapy than the science-dominated thinking in evidence-based practice in psychology. Scientific findings should play a part in psychotherapy. Yet, science is only one among several parameters that are important to understand psychotherapy.

References

Adshead, G. (2018). Security of mind: 20 years of attachment theory and its relevance to psychiatry. *The British Journal of Psychiatry 213*(3), 511–513. http://doi.org/10.1192/bjp.2018.104

American Psychological Association. (2016). Different approaches to psychotherapy. Retrieved from http://www.apa.org/topics/therapy/psychotherapy-approaches.aspx

American Psychological Association. (2017a). Case Example: Jill, a 32-year-old Afghanistan war veteran. Retrieved from https://www.apa.org/ptsd-guideline/resources/cognitive-behavioral-therapy-example

American Psychological Association. (2017b). Ethical principles for psychologists and code of conduct. Retrieved from http://www.apa.org/ethics/code/ethics-code-2017.pdf

Ayer, A. J. (1936). *Language, truth and logic*. London: Penguin books.

Ayer, A. J. (1959). Editor's introduction. In A. J. Ayer (Ed.), *Logical positivism* (pp. 3–28). New York, NY: Free Press.

Beauchamp, T. L. (2003). The nature of applied ethics. In R. G. Frey & C. H. Wellman (Eds.), *A companion to applied ethics* (pp. 1–17). Oxford: Blackwell Publishing.

Beck, A. T. (1976). *Cognitive therapy and the emotional disorders*. New York, NY: International University Press.

Beck, A. T., Epstein, N., Brown, G., & Steer, R. A. (1988a). An inventory for measuring clinical anxiety: Psychometric properties. *Journal of Consulting and Clinical Psychology*, *56*(6), 893–897. http://doi.org/10.1037/0022-006X.56.6.893

Beck, A. T., Steer, R. A., & Carbin, M. G. (1988b). Psychometric properties of the Beck Depression Inventory: Twenty-five years of evaluation. *Clinical Psychology Review*, *8*(1), 77–100. http://doi.org/10.1016/0272-7358(88)90050-5

Beck Institute for Cognitive Behavior Therapy. (2019). History of Cognitive Behavior Therapy. Retrieved from https://beckinstitute.org/about-beck/team/our-history/history-of-cognitive-therapy/

Beck, J. S. (2011). *Cognitive behavior therapy: Basics and beyond* (2nd ed.). New York, NY: Guilford Publications.

Benjamin, C. L., Puleo, C. M., Settipani, C. A., Brodman, D. M., Edmunds, J. M., Cummings, C. M., & Kendall, P. C. (2011). History of cognitive-behavioral therapy in youth. *Child and Adolescent Psychiatric Clinics of North America*, *20*(2), 179–189. http://doi.org/10.1016/j.chc.2011.01.011

Bennet-Levy, J., Westbrook, D., Fennel, M., Cooper, M., Rouf, K., & Hackmann, A. (2004). Behavioural experiments: Historical and conceptual underpinnings. In J. Bennet-Levy, G. Butler, M. Fennel, A. Hackman, M. Mueller, & D. Westbrook (Eds.), *Oxford guide to behavioural experiments in cognitive therapy* (pp. 1–20). Oxford: Oxford University Press.

Bohart, A. C., O'Hara, M., & Leitner, L. M. (1998). Empirically violated treatments: Disenfranchisement of humanistic and other psychotherapies. *Psychotherapy Research*, *8*(2), 141–157. http://doi.org/10.1080/10503309812331332277

Brandchaft, B., & Stolorow, R. D. (1994). The difficult patient. In R. D. Stolorow, G. Atwood, & B. Brandchaft (Eds.), *The intersubjective perspective* (pp. 93–112). New York, NY: Rowman & Littlefield Publishers.

Byrne, P. (2001). Psychiatric stigma. *British Journal of Psychiatry*, *178*(3), 281–284. http://doi.org/10.1192/bjp.178.3.281

Chambless, D. L., & Crits-Christoph, P. (2006). The treatment method In J. C. Norcross, L. E. Beutler, & R. F. Levant (Eds.), *Evidence-based practices in mental health: Debate and dialogue on the fundamental questions*. Washington, DC: American Psychological Association.

Clark, G., & Egan, S. (2015). The Socratic method in cognitive behavioural therapy: A narrative review. *Cognitive Therapy and Research*, *39*(6), 863–879. http://doi.org/10.1007/s10608-015-9707-3

Davies, J. M., & Frawley, M. G. (1991). Dissociative processes and transference-countertransference paradigms in the psychoanalytically oriented treatment of adult survivors of childhood sexual abuse. In S. A. Mitchell & L. Aron (Eds.), *Relational psychoanalysis* (Vol. 14, pp. 269–304). New York, NY: The Analytic Press.

Douglas, H. E. (2009). *Science, policy and the value-free ideal*. Pittsburgh, PA: University of Pittsburgh Press.

Ellis, A. (1962). *Reason and emotion in psychotherapy*. Secaucus, NJ: Lyle Stuart.

Epictetus. (2014). Handbook. In C. Gill (Ed.), *Discourse, fragments, handbook* (pp. 287–348). Oxford: Oxford University Press.

Fernandez-Alvarez, H., Consoli, A. J., & Gomez, B. (2016). Integration in psychotherapy: Reasons and challenges. *American Psychologist*, *71*(8), 820–830. http://doi.org/10.1037/amp0000100

Freud, S. (1961). *The Ego and the Id, and other works* (Vol. 19). London: Hogarth Press and the Institute of Psycho-analysis.

Goldfried, M. R., Burckell, L. A., & Eubanks-Carter, C. (2003). Therapist self-disclosure in cognitive-behavior therapy. *Journal of Clinical Psychology*, *59*(5), 555–568. http://doi.org/10.1002/jclp.10159

Guignon, C. B. (2006). Authenticity, moral values and psychotherapy. In C. B. Guignon (Ed.), *The Cambridge companion to Heidegger* (2nd ed., pp. 268–292). New York, NY: Cambridge University Press.

Hayes, J. A., Gelso, C. J., Goldberg, S., & Kivlighan, D. M. (2018). Countertransference management and effective psychotherapy: Meta-analytic findings. *Psychotherapy*, *55*(4), 496–507. http://doi.org/10.1037/pst0000189

Heidegger, M. (1962). *Being and time*. Oxford: Basil Blackwell.

Hobbs, N. (1948). The development of a code of ethical standards for psychology. *American Psychologist*, *3*(3), 80–84. http://doi.org/10.1037/h0060281

Hume, D. (2009). *A treatise of human nature: Being an attempt to introduce the experimental method of reasoning into moral subjects*. Auckland: The Floating Press.

Husserl, E. (1970). *The crisis of European sciences and transcendental phenomenology: An introduction to phenomenological philosophy*. Evanston, IL: Northwestern University Press.

Jacobsen, B. (2007). *Invitation to existential psychology*. Chichester: John Wiley & Sons.

Kant, I. (1997). *Groundwork of the metaphysics of morals*. Cambridge: Cambridge University Press.

Kierkegaard, S. (1987). *Kierkegaard's writings : 3-4 Pt. 1 : Either/or* (Vol. 3–4, Pt. 1). Princeton, NJ: Princeton University Press.

Lambert, M. J. (2013). Introduction and historical overview. In M. J. Lambert (Eds.), *Bergin and Garfield's handbook of psychotherapy and behaviour change* (pp. 3–20). Hoboken, NJ: John Wiley & Sons.

Latour, B. (1993). *We have never been modern*. New York, NY: Harvester Wheatsheaf.

Lichtenberg, D. D. (2003). Communication in infancy. *Psychoanalytic Inquiry*, *23*(3), 498–520. http://doi.org/10.1080/07351692309349046

Lingiardi, V., & Bornstein, R. F. (2017). Profile of mental functioning. In V. Lingiardi & N. McWilliams (Eds.), *Psychodynamic diagnostic manual* (pp. 75–133). New York, NY: Guilford Press.

Madsen, O. J. (2015). *Optimizing the self : Social representations of self-help*. London: Routledge.

Maroda, K. J. (1991). *The power of countertransference: Innovations in analytic technique*. Chichester: Wiley.

May, R. (1983). *The discovery of being: Writings in existential psychology*. New York, NY: Norton & Company.

McWilliams, N., & Shedler, J. (2017). Personality syndromes. In V. Lingiardi & N. McWilliams (Eds.), *Psychodynamic diagnostic manual* (pp. 15–74). New York, NY: Guilford Press.

Merton, Robert K. (1973). The normative structure of science. In Robert K. Merton (Ed.), *The sociology of science: Theoretical and empirical investigations*. Chicago, IL: University of Chicago Press.

Mitchell, S. A. (2000). *Relationality: From attachment to intersubjectivity* (Vol. 20). New York, NY: The Analytic Press.

Nietzsche, F. (2012). *The Genealogy of Morals*. Newburyport: Dover Publications.

Peirce, C. S., & Jastrow, J. (1884). On Small Differences in Sensation. *Memoirs of the National Academy of Sciences*, *3*, 73–83. Retrieved from http://psychclassics.yorku.ca/Peirce/small-diffs.htm

Pérez-Rojas, A. E., Palma, B., Bhatia, A., Jackson, J., Norwood, E., Hayes, J. A., & Gelso, C. J. (2017). The development and initial validation of the Countertransference Management Scale. *Psychotherapy*, *54*(3), 307–319. http://doi.org/10.1037/pst0000126

Plato. (2010). *Meno & Phaedo*. Cambridge: Cambridge University Press.

Robertson, Donald. (2010). *The philosophy of cognitive-behavioural therapy (CBT): Stoic philosophy as rational and cognitive psychotherapy*. London: Karnac Books.

Robins, C. J., & Block, P. (1989). Cognitive theories of depression viewed from a diathesis-stress perspective: Evaluations of the models of Beck and of Abramson, Seligman, and Teasdale. *Cognitive Therapy and Research*, *13*(4), 29–313. http://doi.org/10.1007/bf01173475

Rorty, R. (1989). *Contingency, irony and solidarity*. New York, NY: Cambridge University Press.

Seligman, M. E., & Csikszentmihalyi, M. (2000). Positive psychology. An introduction. *American Psychologist*, *55*(1), 5–14. http://doi.org/10.1037/0003-066X.55.1.5

Singer, P. (2011). *Practical ethics*. New York, NY: Cambridge University Press.

Stern, D. N. (1985). *The interpersonal world of the infant*. New York, NY: Basic Books.

Stolorow, R. D., & Atwood, G. E. (1992). Three realms of the unconscious. In S. A. Mitchell & L. Aron (Eds.), *Relational psychoanalysis: The emergence of a tradition* (Vol. 14, pp. 365–378). New York, NY: The Analytic Press.

Stricker, G. (2010). *Psychotherapy integration*. Washington, DC: American Psychological Association.

Tillich, P. (1958). *Dynamics of faith*. New York, NY: Harper & Row.

Tjeltveit, A. C. (1999). *Ethics and values in psychotherapy*. London: Routledge.

Tjeltveit, A. C. (2004). The good, the bad, the obligatory, and the virtuous: The ethical contexts of psychotherapy. *Journal of Psychotherapy Integration*, *14*(2), 149–167. http://doi.org/10.1037/1053-0479.14.2.149

Wampold, B. (2001). *The great psychotherapy debate: Models, methods, and findings*. Mahwah, NJ: Lawrence Erlbaum Associates.

Wampold, B. (2011). *Qualities and actions of effective therapists*. Retrieved from https://www.apa.org/education/ce/effective-therapists.pdf:

Wampold, B. (2015). How important are the common factors in psychotherapy? An update. *World Psychiatry*, *14*(3), 270–277. http://doi.org/10.1002/wps.20238

Weinberg, A. M. (1972). Science and trans-science. *Minerva*, *10*(2), 209–222. http://doi.org/10.1007/bf01682418

Winter, D. A. (2013). Still radical after all these years: George Kelly's the psychology of personal constructs. *Clinical Child Psychology and Psychiatry*, *18*(2), 276–283. http://doi.org/10.1177/1359104512454264

6 An ethical demarcation

One of the most important aims of introducing evidence-based practice in psychology was the regulation of practices using psychological knowledge. The policy statement is particularly concerned with regulating psychotherapy. To this aim, evidence-based practice in psychology establishes a demarcation between science and non-science. An example of non-scientific understanding of mental illness is astrology. Astrology's basic tenet is that the motion of faraway heavenly bodies affects people born in a given interval in the calendar. Astrology simply lacks empirical support. Therefore, astrology (to the extent it could be considered psychotherapy) constitutes an illegitimate form of treatment.

The line of demarcation, however, becomes less clear when we compare different treatment forms within established academic psychology. As we have seen, The American Psychological Association operates with five main therapy traditions. These are behavioural therapy, cognitive therapy, psychoanalysis/psychodynamic, humanistic-existential, and eclectic/integrative therapy. Nonetheless, The American Psychological Association have sanctioned a policy statement testing different psychotherapy interventions. Evidence-based practice in psychology ranks different treatment forms according to their empirical status. What is at stake is, of course, the legitimacy of treatment approaches. And more importantly, the well-being of patients.

All forms of regulation of practices involve risk. One risk is that regulatory principles have unintended effects. Therefore, it is crucial that these regulatory principles are subject to analysis uncovering unintended consequences. In the previous chapter, we saw how evidence-based practice in psychology and empirically validated treatments obfuscate our understanding of psychotherapy. The main problem is that it does not include the ethos of psychotherapy. In this chapter, we will focus on how the policy statement for evidence-based practice works as an (implicit) ethical demarcation.

DOI: 10.4324/9781003512141-6

Hidden demarcations

Demarcation is a central concept for understanding some of the most important functions of evidence-based practice in psychology. To demarcate means to separate. Demarcation originally denoted the act of drawing up borders between different states. The term originates from Pope Alexander IV's demarcation of the border between the areas belonging to Spain and Portugal (in the 'New World' in the late 15th century). Later, the term has been deployed by philosopher of science, Karl Popper. It refers to the principles that distinguish science from pseudo-science (Popper, 1963, 2014). The two examples illustrate how a demarcation is normally drawn up by an authority. This authority may be the church, philosophy of science, or a professional association (as is the case with evidence-based practice in psychology).

Evidence-based psychology contains three demarcations: the first is an epistemic demarcation which distinguishes science from non-science. On the one hand, evidence-based practice in psychology rests on a distinction between science-and non-science. As noted in Chapter 4, however, the definition of best evidence is somewhat ambiguous. This indicates tensions in evidence-based practice in psychology. On the one hand, it is crucial for psychologists to base their practice on evidence. On the other, evidence-based practice in psychology does not provide a clear definition of evidence.

The second demarcation distinguishes between good and bad practice. In evidence-based practice in psychology, the relation between these two demarcations is relatively clear-cut. Good practice is based on scientific findings. If there is no scientific support for an intervention, the practice is illegitimate. At the same time, the ideal of best practices in evidence-based practice in psychology also includes other elements. These elements are 'clinical expertise' and 'patients' characteristics, culture, and preferences.' As we will see in Chapter 7, however, these two components are not distinct elements in the policy statement. This entails that evidence-based practice in psychology regulates psychological practice solely based on 'best available research evidence.'

Identifying the epistemic and the practical demarcation is relatively straightforward. They are even included in the title of the policy statement. 'Evidence' indicates an epistemic demarcation and 'practice' indicates a practical demarcation. However, in addition to the epistemic and practical demarcation, there is a third demarcation (Berg, 2019). This demarcation is ethical. The ethical demarcation is, however, not explicit in the policy statement. Nor is it an explicit aim of the policy statement to function as an ethical demarcation. First, it is important to show *that* evidence-based practice in psychology functions as an ethical demarcation. Next, it is important to show *what kind* of ethics it is that regulates psychotherapy. This is the only way to get to the question of whether this regulation may have unintended negative consequences. As the epistemic and the practical demarcation are intertwined with the ethical demarcation, it is, however, worth taking a closer look at these two demarcations.

Epistemic demarcation

An epistemic demarcation sets boundaries for legitimate knowledge. An epistemic demarcation can be drawn on at least two (although related) levels. One is an epistemological level. Epistemology is theory of knowledge. In today's psychology, many different epistemological positions co-exist (Watanabe, 2010). The second level is methodological. It describes the different principles from which we gain empirical knowledge. Psychology is a methodologically pluralistic discipline (Appelbaum et al., 2018; Levitt et al., 2018).

The policy statement (which is built on the concept 'evidence') does not contain explicit epistemological discussions. However, The *Users' Guides to the Medical Literature* (which is considered a key work in evidence-based medicine) does. As we have seen, evidence-based practice in psychology is modelled on evidence-based practice in medicine. Therefore, this work is relevant for understanding evidence-based practice in psychology.

Djulbegovic and Guyatt (2014) discusses the epistemology of evidence-based medicine in a dedicated section in the *Users' Guides to the Medical Literature*. They claim that evidence-based medicine does not profess to present a new medical 'meta-theory.' Nor does it attempt to provide a 'a rigorous epistemological stance' (Djulbegovic & Guyatt, 2014, p. 18) for medical research. Rather, the authors maintain, evidence-based medicine is simply a tool for improving clinical decision-making and problem-solving. It is evidence-based medicine's foundation in medical research that ensures best practice. Therefore, it is interesting that the authors also claim that:

> [a]pproaches to scientific inquiry [...] depend on how one views the nature of knowledge as evidence. How it should be acquired, and how it should be applied (epistemology).
>
> (Djulbegovic & Guyatt, 2014, p. 16)

On the one hand, the authors want to avoid epistemology and 'meta-theory.' On the other, they claim that these issues are crucial.

Djulbegovic and Guyatt (2014) present two concepts to position evidence-based medicine. These two concepts are 'evidentialism' and 'reliabilism.' Although Djulbegovic and Guyatt do not claim to represent an epistemological position, the two concepts nonetheless have an epistemological function. Evidentialism states that a belief's validity is proportional to the evidence supporting it. Here, evidence refers to the data used in support of a statement. One example could be the statement 'cognitive-behavioural therapy is an effective treatment for depression.' This statement is supported if evidence (typically qua randomised controlled trials) indicates that cognitive-behavioural therapy is an effective treatment form for depression. Epistemology, in contrast, is theory of knowledge. Epistemology cannot be justified by knowledge itself. Djulbegovic and Guyatt presuppose that epistemic value which epistemology establishes. Thus, their argument is circular.

Djulbegovic and Guyatt (2014) second concept, 'reliabilism,' indicates that best evidence is produced by the most reliable knowledge processes (note, the difference from the use of the term 'reliabilism' discussed in Chapter 8). It is trivially true that knowledge achieved through reliable processes is preferable to knowledge achieved through non-reliable processes. The question remains, however, what constitutes a reliable process. Djulbegovic and Guyatt (2014) do not address this issue. Upon closer scrutiny, then, evidence-based medicine is not well founded. Evidentialism and reliabilism are not (satisfactory) epistemological positions. Consequently, evidence-based medicine (and evidence-based practice in psychology) lacks an epistemological basis.

The epistemic demarcation in evidence-based practice in psychology is based on methodology. The policy statement addresses the complementary strengths and weaknesses of different methods and designs. As seen in Chapter 4, it is unclear whether evidence-based practice in psychology has a strict methodological hierarchy. On the one hand, several different research designs and methods are acknowledged. On the other, there is an explicit methodological hierarchy for specific interventions (and a less formal hierarchy, implied in the descriptions of the different methods). Ultimately, randomised controlled trials hold a privileged position, although less pronounced than in evidence-based medicine.

The epistemic demarcation in evidence-based practice in psychology, then, is epistemologically unfounded and methodologically vague. Thomas Kuhn has provided some of the most well-known descriptions of science. According to Kuhn, parts of scientific practices are based on habit. Such depictions do not reflect normative ideals such as critical thinking and rationality (Kuhn, 2012). It may, however, seem like Kuhn's characteristic of science resonates well with evidence-based practice in psychology. It lacks a solid foundation and the clarity of rational argumentation.

The practical demarcation: What works…

The second demarcation in evidence-based practice in psychology is practical. After the advent of evidence-based practice in psychology, the phrase 'that works' gained popularity. It is a rhetorically potent expression.

Previously, it was simply assumed that certain treatment forms were effective. Now, through empirical testing, we *know* that these treatment forms work in practice. The practical demarcation in evidence-based practice in psychology is, however, somewhat ambiguous. Evidence-based practice in psychology is founded on an ideal consisting of three components: 'best available research evidence,' 'clinical expertise,' and 'patient's culture, characteristics, and preferences.' The ideal for best practices, in other words, contains more than 'best available research evidence.' As we will see in Chapter 7, the attempt to distinguish the three components has not been successful. This means that it actually consists of *one* component: 'best available research evidence.'

The component 'best available research evidence' differentiates between the theoretical and practical value of research through two quality parameters. Efficacy denotes the robustness of the scientific findings. Effectiveness indicates how well interventions work in practice. The practical value of research is reflected in the parameter effectiveness. Evidence-based practice in psychology intends to regulate the application of psychological knowledge. For a psychologist who wants to use knowledge in a clinical situation, there is really only *one* relevant question, which is, whether it can contribute to the realisation of some defined aims. If the knowledge can contribute to realising these aims, it has practical value (Berg, 2021). A strong scientific base for a treatment does not make much of a practical if it turns out that the treatment is ineffective. As evidence normally is general while treatment normally is individual, this distinction is significant.

Theoretical ghosts

The Scottish philosopher Alasdair MacIntyre (1929–) has unveiled 'theoretical ghosts' in modern administration. Although many practitioners assume they are simply doing 'what works,' their actions generally reflect some moral or ethical presuppositions. According to MacIntyre, one of the most important functions of ethical analyses is to uncover such 'theoretical ghosts.' This is the only way to address the underlying ethical principles and, if need be, refute them (MacIntyre, 2011).

MacIntyre (2011) argues that 'theoretical ghosts' thrive in Weberian bureaucracies. They simply aim towards implementing pre-defined goals optimally (MacIntyre, 2011). Hence, cost-benefit analysis is a much-used tool in modern Weberian bureaucracies. Cost-benefit analyses were invented to assess means to pre-defined ends. They compare the expected costs and benefits of different alternatives. The best course of action provides the most benefit per cost. Both costs and benefits are 'expected,' that is, based on probability estimates. Thus, there are risks of errors in the analyses which can deviate from actual benefits (Adler, 2015; Adler &

Posner, 1999; Frank, 2000; Harvey, Camasso, & Jagannathan, 2004; Lowry & Peterson, 2011; Sen, 2000).

A fairly straightforward way to identify effective means is to conduct randomised controlled trials (and add cost-estimations) (Polsky & Glick, 2009). Randomised controlled trials are, in other words, a useful tool for conducting cost-benefit analyses in Weberian bureaucracies. At the same time, the combination may obscure the purpose of a service. Differences that are not illuminated in bureaucratic assessments (i.e., cost-benefit analyses) may still profoundly impact services. One example, which will be addressed below, is a technology-mediated psychotherapy service called 'internet-based guided self-help therapy.' Depending on the assessment parameters, internet-based guided self-help therapy is deemed a more or less adequate alternative to traditional face-to-face therapy.

Ethics and evidence-based practice

C.P. Snow's (1905–1980) classic essay 'The Two Cultures' can shed light on the general absence of critical analysis of evidence-based practice in psychology. In the text, C.P. Snow depicted two distinct academic cultures. On the one hand you find the literary intellectuals (typically, humanistic scholars). On the other you find the scientists (typically, qua natural scientists). C.P. Snow claimed that there was very little interaction between the two cultures. At the same time, quite a few academic problems transcend established disciplinary boundaries. Therefore, isolated academic communities often contribute to fragmentation of knowledge, and a lack of holistic understanding of a range of phenomena and societal challenges (Snow, 1993).

Woolfolk describes a similar division in psychotherapy. On the one hand, some psychotherapists adhere to humanistic knowledge criteria. These are typically found within the humanist/existential tradition and partly within the psychoanalytic/psychodynamic tradition. On the other, we find psychotherapists oriented towards natural sciences. These are typically associated with cognitive and behavioural psychology. The two camps typically differ in their assessment of evidence-based practice in psychology. For many humanistic psychotherapists, evidence-based practice in psychology is obviously fallacious (Bohart, O'Hara, & Leitner, 1998). For psychotherapists associated with natural sciences, it is obviously necessary (Lilienfeld, McKay, & Hollon, 2018; Lilienfeld, Ritschel, Lynn, Cautin, & Latzman, 2014). According to Woolfolk (2015), there has been little interaction between these two camps. At times, straw man arguments have been used to ascribe non-representative opinions to the opponents.

If there are relatively distinct academic cultures in psychotherapy, it is not unthinkable that they have different criteria for assessing quality. A study conducted by Walfish, McAlister, O'Donnell, and Lambert

(2012) found that most psychotherapists consider themselves to be better than their peers. No one assessed themselves as below average, and only 8,4% below the 75th percentile. The average self-assessment was around the 80th percentile (Walfish et al., 2012). People's inclination to overestimate their own skills and performances is well documented. Self-serving bias refers to our inclination to interpret events to our benefit (Shepperd, Malone, & Sweeny, 2008). To some extent at least, the findings of Walfish et al. (2012) may be explained by a 'self-serving bias.' Nonetheless, Woolfolk (2015) asks whether such findings may also indicate that psychotherapists differ in their perceptions of what psychotherapy is. To be able to assess whether an act or an intervention is good, it must be related to a normative standard. As we have seen, there are different (often implicit) normative standards constituting various psychotherapy schools. This means that the parameters and criteria of assessment also vary (across these psychotherapy schools). However, the same pertains to the policy statement *in toto*. The policy statement (itself) is based on some normative criteria defining 'goodness.'

Evidence-based practice in psychology as utilitarianism

There is a third demarcation in evidence-based practice in psychology (Berg, 2019). This demarcation functions as an implicit ethical demarcation. As evidence-based practice in psychology claims to provide a demarcation between legitimate and illegitimate psychological practice, the ethical demarcation obscures the range of relevant ethical perspectives. As a result, we are left with fewer ethical resources for assessing psychotherapy. In a complex practice like psychotherapy, however, a range of different ethical theories are relevant.

The ethical demarcation in evidence-based practice in psychology is utilitarian, which is one of the main traditions in normative ethics. This is not a uniform tradition, but it is possible to sketch some typical features:

- Utility: Goodness is defined by utility (e.g., the presence of pleasure and the absence of pain).
- Consequentialist: Judging the goodness of actions by their consequences.
- Universalist: All (affected) parties should have an equal priority.
- Aggregationist: The goodness of outcomes is determined by aggregated outcomes.

Many regard the British philosopher Jeremy Bentham (1748–1832) as the founder of utilitarianism. According to Bentham, 'the good' is consequences that maximises hedonistic pleasure and minimises pain. The best action could be identified through a calculus that combines different factors (Bentham, 1781). John Stuart Mill (1806–1873) is another well-known utilitarian. Although Mill (1991) distinguishes between bodily pleasure (e.g., eating candy) and more active and higher forms of pleasure (e.g., reading a novel), he subscribed to the 'greatest happiness principle':

> actions are right in proportion as they tend to promote happiness, wrong as they tend to produce the reverse of happiness. By happiness is intended pleasure, and the absence of pain; by unhappiness, pain, and the privation of pleasure.
>
> (p. 137)

Evidence-based practice in psychology claims to provide the best treatment because it is based on scientific evidence. Hence, it reflects the ethical relevance of standardised measurements found in utilitarianism. In evidence-based practice in psychology, randomised controlled trials are deemed particularly informative. Randomised controlled trials examine the consequences of different alternatives (i.e., treatment effectiveness). This reflects utilitarian consequentialism. The typical effects sought are symptom reduction (entailing that pain is reduced and pleasure is increased). Depression can serve as an example. Some of the symptoms of depression include the lack of ability to experience joy, a feeling of hopelessness, lack of appetite, and extensive self-criticism. Reducing these symptoms would, in other words, contribute to the reduction of pain and the increment of pleasure. The same generally applies to the reduction of symptoms across mental illnesses. In addition, randomised controlled trials test groups. When this knowledge is applied in clinical practice, it is universalistic in the sense that all patients with a given diagnosis are treated equally. If randomised controlled trials suggest that cognitive-behavioural therapy is most effective in treating phobia, then an evidence-based practitioner would use that treatment method for all patients.

J.J.C. Smart (1920–2012) argued that one should identify the preferred action through probability calculations (echoing Bentham). J.J.C. Smart launched an ethical distinction. Let's start by taking an example. An analysis might indicate that there is an 85% probability that an intervention will lead to a given outcome. Of course, a practitioner might intervene in accordance with this knowledge, but fail to produce the expected outcome. To clarify this difference, J.J.C. Smart introduced the distinction between rational and good actions. An action is rational if we have good reason to believe that it will result in good consequences. Good actions, however, must result in actual good consequences. We may act rationally on the bases of scientific knowledge, without ending up with good clinical actions (Smart, 1973).

However, there is a problem with J.J.C. Smart's (1973) quantification of ethics. Psychotherapy is highly complex. It is difficult to establish whether a clinical action has a given effect. J.J.C. Smart's (1973) ideal entails that we must know *all relevant* outcomes of a given intervention. In the case of psychotherapy, this is an exceedingly high number of outcomes. What is more, scientific conclusions are seldom unequivocal. For this reason, it is very difficult to determine what would be a rational choice of action based on scientific data. The distinction between rational and good outcomes only adds to the problem.

There is yet another relevant distinction between act utilitarianism and rule utilitarianism. Act utilitarianism defines the good as the singular actions that result in the greatest possible amount of utility. Rule utilitarianism defines the good as the rules that result in the greatest possible amount of utility. We can imagine a situation where terrorists have taken hostages and demand a ransom. In such a situation, act utilitarianists might argue that one should pay the ransom to free the hostages. Rule utilitarianists might, on the other hand, argue that paying ransoms in hostage situations will lead to an increment of such incidents. Therefore, the best rule for action would be to 'pay no ransom.'

The distinction between act utilitarianism and rule utilitarianism is relevant for evidence-based practice in psychology. Anjum and Mumford (2016) claimed that evidence-based practice is rule utilitarian. Research evidence from randomised controlled trials inform action on group level. Thus, it is rule utilitarian. However, Anjum and Mumford (2016) argued that treatment is (at least typically) individual. Thus, while evidence-based practice is act utilitarian, treating individual patients should be act utilitarian. The evidence, which is general, must always be adapted to a patient, who is an individual (Anjum & Mumford, 2016).

Philosopher Bernard Williams (1929–2003) argued that while utilitarianism does not necessarily arrive at the wrong conclusion, it makes us act without adequate reflection. Thus, we might fail to develop as ethical agents (Williams, 1973). A complex practice such as psychotherapy requires extensive ethical reflection. It is insufficient to simply narrow ethical concerns down to utility. To illustrate this point, we will take a closer look at internet-based guided self-help. This example will be discussed in the light of three non-utilitarian ethical positions which are marginalised in evidence-based practice in psychology.

Internet-based guided self-help

Psychotherapy has traditionally taken place between two (or more) people who are in the same room. As new information technologies have emerged, however, such technologies have been tested for psychotherapeutic purposes. This has resulted in internet-based guided self-help. Internet-based guided self-help is employed in healthcare as an alternative to face-to-face therapy.

There is a distinction between pure self-help and guided self-help. In pure self-help, the patient undertakes a treatment programme without support from a professional practitioner. Conversely, in guided self-help, the patient is supported by a professional practitioner. Nonetheless, the treatment is largely based on the patient's efforts. There are a range of ways of providing guidance in guided self-help. One may, for instance, provide guidance face to face, over the telephone, or through the internet (Andersson et al., 2008; Lindefors & Andersson, 2016). Internet is, however, the probably the most accessible and cost-effective alternative.

Neither the idea of technology-mediated psychotherapy nor self-help programmes are new. A well-known example of technology-mediated psychotherapy is the software ELIZA. ELIZA was developed to simulate Rogerian therapy. Hence, it 'mirrored' the patient responses. At the time, the intention, notably, was to demonstrate the limitations of computer software (Weizenbaum, 1966). Although the software has become more sophisticated since ELIZA, there are still obvious limitations to what a computer can achieve when it comes to a more general understanding of a (clinical) situation (Mitchell, 2019). A general understanding is typically needed in psychotherapy.

Medical and psychotherapeutic self-help pamphlets have been distributed for some time. In 1969, former president of the American Psychological Association, George Miller, encouraged psychologists to 'give psychology away.' He wanted to help patients to help themselves instead of receiving help through healthcare professionals (Banyard & Hulme, 2015). With the proliferation of the internet, it became possible to spread information more effectively. This has led to an increased interest in exploring the cost-efficiency of internet-mediated psychotherapy.

There are guided self-help programmes for different schools of psychotherapy (Johansson et al., 2012; Ly et al., 2014). Notwithstanding, the basic template of internet-based guided self-help is probably most commensurable with cognitive-behavioural therapy. This school normally operates with patient tasks and 'home-work,' even in face-to-face versions (Freeman, 2007). In internet-based guided self-help, the patient is typically guided through various modules. The different modules lead the patient through different steps which contain different tasks. The modules contain information about the most significant techniques and mechanisms for change within the psychotherapy school in question. They also contain common challenges and problems that tend to occur in treatment. The main goal is that patients acquire skills and knowledge to be able to help themselves. The therapist supports and guides the patient towards this aim. It is relatively common to have some follow-ups of symptoms through questionnaires (Nordgreen et al., 2010; Stott et al., 2013).

According to the research literature, there is a difference between the effectiveness of pure and guided self-help therapy. Pure self-help therapy is not very effective. In contrast, guided self-help is on par with face-to-face therapy effectiveness and cost-efficiency (Cuijpers, Donker, van Straten, Li, & Andersson, 2010). As treatment may be offered across great geographical areas, the potential cost-efficiency is high, particularly, in countries or regions with a scattered and dispersed population. The same goes for forms of therapy which are more manual based and which therefore require a less broad competence on the part of the therapist (Cuijpers et al., 2010; Seekles, van Straten, Beekman, van Marwijk, & Cuijpers, 2011).

If one follows utilitarian principles, guided self-help is a rational treatment choice. The classical utilitarian postulate is the greatest benefit for the greatest number of people. If utility in this context is the reduction of symptoms, and if the greatest possible reduction is represented by cost-efficiency, we see that internet-based guided self-help is well suited for a utilitarian schema. At the same time, a range of other ethical issues are relevant when assessing psychotherapy. These may illuminate other issues marginalised by the ethical demarcation in evidence-based practice in psychology. Below, three different alternative ethical perspectives will be addressed: Foucault's discursive ethics, phenomenological ethics, and virtue ethics. These perspectives represent other approaches to understanding *inter alia* the implicit premises upon which different forms of practice rest, and the relationship between science and practice.

Foucauldian ethics

One of Michel Foucault's (1926–84) major contributions was the analyses of the conditions of possibility for knowledge. The conditions of possibility determine possible bodies of scientific knowledge. In the history of philosophy, such preconditions have typically been tied to the human cognitive and sensory apparatus (Kant, 2009). Therefore, one has tended to see these preconditions as invariable and universal. Foucault, however, problematised the idea that such stable, ahistorical preconditions exist. He points to the history of science (and philosophy) to support this claim. If one looks at the history of the human or life sciences (e.g., economics, biology, psychology), certain patterns emerge. According to Foucault, these disciplines have more continuity across disciplinary boundaries (at a given point in time) than they have within a discipline across historical periods. He saw this as indicative of the existence of historically variable preconditions structuring scientific knowledge. Another central point in Foucault's analyses is that the historical agents are often unaware of these preconditions. This means that scientific knowledge is contingent on rules of knowledge which is generally obscure. Herein lies one of the most important ethical points of Foucault's analyses: as these preconditions for knowledge shape knowledge itself, analyses of the preconditions for knowledge may help us identify problematic aspects of knowledge production and the practical use of knowledge.

This point is illustrated in Foucault's text *Madness and civilization*. In *Madness and civilization*, Foucault showed how 'madness' (a deliberately provocative term) has been understood in various historical periods (Foucault, 1977). He described three distinct historical periods to illustrate the variation in the conception of 'madness.' These historical periods are the Renaissance, the classical age, and Modernity (here, a different time interval from the 'modernity' discussed in Chapter 2). In the Renaissance, madness was connected to life's futility. 'The mad' shares the characteristics of the 'Shakespearian fool.' The 'Shakespearian fool' is both odd and wise, offering an original perspective. The insights of 'the mad' are connected to the tragic dimensions of life and most notably the finitude of life. In the Renaissance, 'the mad' are partly integrated to society. However, Foucault argued that around 1650, there was an abrupt shift in the understanding of madness. Over a short period, a significant proportion of Paris' population was locked up. This signalled the emergence of a new understanding of madness in the classical age. Madness became a threat to social order itself, and therefore, it was crucial to lock up 'the mad.' Furthermore, 'the mad' were understood as humans devoid of their humanity. This conception resulted in deeply inhuman practices where humans were treated as animals. However, 'madness' was not seen as a problem that could be solved through knowledge. It was exclusively a moral issue. The later reformers of the subsequent modern era, such as Phillipe Pinel (1745–1826) and Samuel Tuke (1784–1857), wanted to humanise treatment. These reformers brought patients out of the asylum and treated them in the clinic (exempting physical violence). By the same token, Foucault noted that Pinel and Tuke dominated their patients in subtle ways. For instance, it was not uncommon for patients to have to mimic the bourgeoise in simulated tea parties. The idea was to re-introduce the patients to a 'healthy, bourgeois' way of life (Foucault, 2001).

In his later thinking, Foucault analysed the relationship between knowledge and power. In one of his most famous texts, *Discipline and punish*, Foucault analysed how modern institutions are the result of historical contingencies. These contingencies shape both the understanding of ourselves and others. One of the main points in this work is that the prison has become the paradigmatic modern institution. Foucault describes the modern society as panoptic. In the panoptic society, one cannot tell whether one is being observed or not. Hence, one must internalise an observer's standards and act 'as if' one is observed at all times. This entails far more subtle forms of discipline than those of previous societies. In these societies, the mechanisms of control were more visible, and at times quite spectacular, but more limited in their scope (Foucault, 1977).

Foucault's thinking may help us identify other facets of internet-based guided self-help. Through internet-based guided self-help, patients are construed in new ways. The treatment is no longer located in out-patient clinics, but largely takes place in the patient's home (and natural environment). Patients are encouraged to make a weekly schedule to integrate the interventions with everyday activities. One risk is that the identity as a patient consolidates because the boundaries between the clinic and everyday life become vaguer. Through the course of the treatment, the patient's symptoms are monitored by a healthcare professional. In this way, internet-based guided self-help treatment encompasses an extent of surveillance and self-monitoring not typically found in conventional face-to-face therapy. This aspect is even more prevalent when it comes to the cultivation of the patient's own ability to complete the treatment and prevent relapse. This practice is problematic if social causes are (erroneously) attributed to the individual patient. One example could be a situation in which a patient is held responsible for mental illness caused by an unhealthy work environment.

One of the most important rationales for guided self-help is accessibility. In principle, anyone who has access to communication technology can receive guided self-help. Accessibility is, however, not an unqualified benefit in healthcare services. More accessible healthcare services entail a greater disease-awareness (both for the individual and the society at large). If accessibility generates an overly extensive focus on disease, it may itself generate more suffering. The term for such a development is medicalisation (Lupton, 1997; Maturo, 2012). It is of ethical importance to pay attention to such developments, not the least when technological fixes become ever more sophisticated and accessible.

Phenomenological ethics

A basic premise of phenomenological thinking is that knowledge (including science) must be connected to human experience (Merleau-Ponty, 2004). As already noted, Edmund Husserl described a crisis in the understanding of science. After the Scientific Revolution, some turn to scientific models for descriptions of the world in full. Husserl (1970), in contrast, argued that our lifeworld is primordial and forms the conditions of possibility for scientific models. The lifeworld is our everyday interaction with the phenomena that constitute the background for any understanding (including scientific models). Hence, any substantial understanding of a scientific object must include this background (Husserl, 1970).

This is one of the main points in Heidegger's phenomenology. In *Being and Time* (1962), he outlines the lifeworld in some detail. Heidegger's point of departure is a critique of Cartesian philosophy. Descartes holds that the world consists of two types of substance. The first is a 'thinking substance' or human consciousness. The second is matter, which constitutes the objects in the world (i.e., anything with extension). Heidegger, on the other hand, claimed that subject and object are intertwined. Thus, a new concept is needed. Heidegger coins it *Dasein* which emphasises the interconnectedness of humans and the world (*da* means 'there' and *sein* means 'being'). Humans have some structures that provide the structures for our existence (i.e., the existentials). Two structures are of particular interest here. One is that we are deeply relational beings (we are 'with-beings'). The other is that we care about our own existence and that we have practical projects carried out for some purpose or ultimate concern (Heidegger, 1962).

The French philosopher Emmanuel Levinas (1906–1995) developed Heidegger's phenomenology. While Heidegger did emphasise human relationality, Levinas radicalised this aspect of his thinking. According to Levinas, 'The Other' constitutes the meaning webs through which we understand the world. This includes our very perception and the language we use to describe it. This realisation pervades Levinas' ethics. As relationally constituted beings, the most urgent ethical commitment is to care for the vulnerability of 'The Other.' This is most clearly experienced when encountering the face of 'The Other.' At the same time, 'The Other' is unfathomable. This, in turn, requires humility in encounters with other human beings and even more so when we try to help people suffering from mental illnesses (Gantt, 2000; Levinas, 1972).

In internet-based guided self-help therapy, the experience that calls us to help other human-beings is marginalised. The interaction takes place by means of technology where the patient interacts directly with the software and communicates with a therapist through the chat-function. As empirical research has shown that the therapeutic alliance is an important ingredient in good treatment, the therapeutic alliance is reconceptualised as a 'relationship' between the patient and the software program. The 'therapeutic alliance' is typically conceptualised as the affective bond between therapist and patient, the agreement on the methods and agreement on the end goal of the treatment (Horvath & Bedi, 2002). In internet-based guided self-help, the alliance is surveyed through a questionnaire. This indicates an expectation that a human's relation to other humans is comparable to a human's relation to a machine (Gómez Penedo et al., 2019). However, research on artificial intelligence does not provide much support for such an idea (Mitchell, 2019). From the point of view of phenomenological ethics, this is ethically problematic (Levinas, 1972).

Internet-based guided self-help does not incorporate the fundamental humility in phenomenological ethics. Internet-based guided self-help often addresses a patient group. Such recommendations may be more or less compatible with the needs of an individual in distress. Thus, ethical resources are needed to highlight this aspect and utilitarianism is generally not very well suited for this purpose.

Moreover, internet-based guided self-help is symptomatic for a widespread perception of humans in industrialised societies. In his later works, Heidegger (1953) described the current era as the 'age of technology.' In the age of technology, all things are resources to be used. This does not only apply to objects, but ultimately even to human beings. As humans have become measurable resources (comparable to other resources), their health may also be included in calculi and compared to other goods or evils (Heidegger, 1973, 2002). Internet-based guided self-help resonates the understanding of humans as a resource because psychotherapy becomes de-personified. Alternatively, therapeutic work could focus more on the human encounter and to identify solutions to the individual problems of the individual patient. In such a therapeutic practice, the humanism of the patient is re-established as a core principle of treatment.

Virtue ethics

Virtue ethics originated in Ancient Greece (MacIntyre, 1967). In *The Republic*, Plato (1993) described the development of good character and how it is inextricably connected to the development of a good society. In *Nicomachean Ethics*, Aristotle (385–323 BC) addresses similar topics. Virtue ethics define 'the good' by the source of the action. In other words, 'the good' are character traits enabling the actor to realise some good outcome relatively consistently. In that sense, it is also consequentialist (like utilitarianism). Virtue ethics is central in Chapter 8, which addresses integration in evidence-based practice in psychology.

A central topic in *Nicomachean Ethics* is the relationship between knowledge and practice. To clarify this relationship, Aristotle describes three different kinds of knowledge. *Episteme* denotes (non-practical) theoretical knowledge (such as pure mathematics or logic). *Techne* is the knowledge of how to produce certain standardised artefacts or end results. Some examples are the construction of an object and practical routines for hygiene at a hospital. A third kind of knowledge, which is particularly relevant for psychotherapy, is *phronesis* or practical wisdom. Practical wisdom is not merely knowledge about means, but also to assess aims. It is the kind of knowledge that enables an individual to select good aims in a given situation. In determining what outcomes that are good or bad, our thinking must include context, because what is *actually* good or bad is always context dependent. For example, to be untruthful is normally wrong. However, an exception would be protecting a child from learning about the cruelties of the world. It is normally wrong not to return something you have borrowed from a friend, but not if the object may harm the owner of the object or someone else.

Internet-based guided self-help conceptualises psychotherapy as *techne*. The assumption is that the categorisation of different patients and scientific knowledge about effectiveness suffices for good psychotherapeutic treatment of individual patients. Internet-based guided self-help treatment is often relatively structured. Thus, there is a low degree of individual adaption. This is problematic considering the major importance of individual difference in psychotherapy. It is a particularly pressing concern when it comes to the issue of patient autonomy.

Virtue ethics emphasise the importance of individualisation. Individualisation requires several different sources of information. One of the problems with internet-based guided self-help is that it provides less information than face-to-face psychotherapy. Information about the patient's body movements, speaking rate, attire, spontaneous outbursts are just some examples that may provide information for tailoring treatment. In a practice such as psychotherapy, the goals are often individual. The practice ultimately revolves around creating a better life for an individual. Hence, an important aspect of psychotherapy is marginalised in internet-based guided self-help therapy.

Conclusion

Although evidence-based practice in psychology was launched as an epistemic and practical demarcation, it also functions as an ethical demarcation. The ethical demarcation is structured by utilitarian principles. Delimiting the assessment of psychotherapy intervention to utilitarian parameters reduces the number of available resources for making good ethical judgements of and within psychotherapeutic practice. Psychotherapy is a complex practice. It is untenable to let a specific kind of ethics regulate it (and not the less implicitly). The main point is not that utilitarianism is a normative ethical tradition with no relevance for psychotherapy (because it clearly has). The problem is that it has been allowed to take the position as supreme normative ethical tradition although this was never a stated intention.

References

Adler, M. D. (2015). Value and cost-benefit analysis. In I. Hirose & J. Olson (Eds.), *The Oxford handbook of value theory* (pp. 317–337). New York, NY: Oxford University Press.

Adler, M. D., & Posner, E. A. (1999). Rethinking cost-benefit analysis. *The Yale Law Journal*, *109*(2), 165–247. http://doi.org/10.1086/428461

Andersson, G., Bergström, J., Buhrman, M., Carlbring, P., Holländare, F., Kaldo, V., … Waara, J. (2008). Development of a new approach to guided self-help via the internet: The Swedish experience. *Journal of*

Technology in Human Services, *26*(2–4), 161–181. http://doi.org/10.1080/15228830802094627

Anjum, R. L., & Mumford, S. D. (2016). A philosophical argument against evidence-based policy. *Journal of Evaluation in Clinical Practice*, 1045–1050. http://doi.org/10.1111/jep.12578

Appelbaum, M., Cooper, H., Kline, R. B., Evan, M.-W., Nezu, A. M., and Rao, S. M. (2018). Journal article reporting standards for quantitative research in psychology: The APA Publications and Communications Board task force report. *American Psychologist*, *73*(1), 3–25.

Banyard, P., & Hulme, J. E. (2015). Giving psychology away: How George Miller's vision is being realised by psychological literacy. *Psychology Teaching Review*, *21*(2), 93–101.

Bentham, Jeremy (1781). *An introduction to the principles of morals and legislation*. Kitchener: Batoche Books. http://socserv2.socsci.mcmaster.ca/econ/ugcm/3ll3/bentham/morals.pdf.

Berg, H. (2019). How does evidence-based practice in psychology work? – As an ethical demarcation. *Philosophical Psychology*, *32*(6), 855–875. http://doi.org/10.1080/09515089.2019.1632424

Berg, H. (2021). Why only efficiency, and not efficacy, matters in psychotherapy practice. *Frontiers in Psychology*, *12*. http://doi.org/10.3389/fpsyg.2021.603211

Bohart, A. C., O'Hara, M., & Leitner, L. M. (1998). Empirically violated treatments: Disenfranchisement of humanistic and other psychotherapies. *Psychotherapy Research*, *8*(2), 141–157. http://doi.org/10.1080/10503309812331332277

Cuijpers, P., Donker, T., van Straten, A., Li, J., & Andersson, G. (2010). Is guided self-help as effective as face-to-face psychotherapy for depression and anxiety disorders? A systematic review and meta-analysis of comparative outcome studies. *Psychological medicine*, *40*(12), 1943–1957. http://doi.org/10.1017/S0033291710000772

Djulbegovic, B., & Guyatt, G. (2014). Evidence-based medicine and the theory of knowledge. In G. Guyatt, D. Rennie, M. O. Meade, & D. J. Cook (Eds.), *User's guides to the medical literature* (pp. 15–19). New York, NY: McGraw-Hill.

Foucault, M. (1977). *Discipline and punish: The birth of the prison*. London: Allen Lane.

Foucault, M. (2001). *Madness and civilization: A history of insanity in the age of reason*. London: Routledge.

Frank, R. H. (2000). Why is cost-benefit analysis so controversial? *The Journal of Legal Studies*, *29*(S2), 913–930. http://doi.org/10.1086/468099

Freeman, A. (2007). The use of homework in cognitive behavior therapy: Working with complex anxiety and insomnia. *Cognitive and Behavioral Practice*, *14*(3), 261–267. http://doi.org/10.1016/j.cbpra.2006.10.005

Gantt, E. E. (2000). Levinas, psychotherapy, and the ethics of suffering. *Journal of Humanistic Psychology*, *40*(3), 9–28. http://doi.org/10.1177/0022167800403002

Gómez Penedo, J. M., Berger, T., Holtforth, M., Krieger, T., Schröder, J., Hohagen, F., … Klein, J. P. (2019). The Working Alliance Inventory for guided Internet interventions (WAI-I). *Journal of Clinical Psychology*, 1–14. http://doi.org/10.1002/jclp.22823

Harvey, C., Camasso, M. J., & Jagannathan, R. (2004). Conducting cost-benefit analysis in human services setting. In A. R. Roberts & K. R. Yeager (Eds.), *Evidence-based practice manual: Research and outcome measures in health and human services*. New York, NY: Oxford University Press.

Heidegger, M. (1953). The question concerning technology. In David Farrell Krell (ed.), *Heidegger: Basic writings*. London: Routledge.

Heidegger, M. (1962). *Being and time, Sein und Zeit*. Oxford: Basil Blackwell.

Heidegger, M. (2002). The age of the world picture. In J. Young and K Haynes (Eds.), *Off the beaten track* (pp. 57–86). Cambridge: Cambridge University Press.

Horvath, A. O., & Bedi, R. P. (2002). The alliance. In J. C. Norcross (Ed.), *Psychotherapy relationships that work: Therapist contributions and responsiveness to patients* (pp. 37–70). New York, NY: Oxford University Press.

Husserl, E. (1970). *The crisis of european sciences and transcendental phenomenology: An introduction to phenomenological philosophy*. Evanston, IL: Northwestern University Press.

Johansson, R., Ekbladh, S., Hebert, A., Lindström, M., Möller, S., Petitt, E., … Andersson, G. (2012). Psychodynamic guided self-help for adult depression through the internet: A randomised controlled trial. *PloS one*, *7*(5), e38021–e38021. http://doi.org/10.1371/journal.pone.0038021

Kant, I. (2009). *The critique of pure reason*. Auckland: The Floating Press.

Kuhn, Thomas. (2012). *The structure of scientific revolutions* (4 ed). Chicago, IL: University of Chicago Press.

Levinas, E. (1972). *The humanism of the Other*. Chicago, IL: University of Illinois Press.

Levitt, H. M., Bamberg, M., Creswell, J. W., Frost, D. M., Josselson, R., & Suárez-Orozco, C. (2018). Journal article reporting standards for qualitative primary, qualitative meta-analytic, and mixed methods research in psychology: The APA Publications and Communications Board task force report. *American Psychologist*, *73*(1). https://doi.org/10.1037/amp0000151

Lilienfeld, S. O., McKay, D., & Hollon, S. D. (2018). Why randomised controlled trials of psychological treatments are still essential. *The Lancet Psychiatry*, *5*(7), 536–538. http://doi.org/10.1016/S2215-0366(18)30045-2

Lilienfeld, S. O., Ritschel, L. A., Lynn, S. J., Cautin, R. L., & Latzman, R. D. (2014). Why ineffective psychotherapies appear to work: A taxonomy of causes of spurious therapeutic effectiveness. *Perspectives on Psychological Science*, *9*(4), 355–387. http://doi.org/10.1177/1745691614535216

Lindefors, N., & Andersson, G. (2016). *Guided internet-based treatments in psychiatry* (1. ed.). Gram: Springer

Lowry, R., & Peterson, M. (2011). Cost-benefit analysis and non-utilitarian ethics. *Politics, Philosophy & Economics*, *11*(3), 258–279. http://doi.org/10.1177/1470594X11416767

Lupton, D. (1997). Foucault and the medicalisation critique. In A. R. Petersen & R. Bunton (Eds.), *Foucault, health and medicine* (pp. 94–113). London: Routledge.

Ly, K. H., Trüschel, A., Jarl, L., Magnusson, S., Windahl, T., Johansson, R., … Andersson, G. (2014). Behavioural activation versus mindfulness-based guided self-help treatment administered through a smartphone application: A randomised controlled trial. *BMJ Open*, *4*(1), e003440. http://doi.org/10.1136/bmjopen-2013-003440

MacIntyre, A. (1967). *A short history of ethics*. London: Routledge & Kegan Paul.

Maturo, A. (2012). Medicalization: Current concept and future directions in a bionic society. *Mens Sana Monographs*, *10*(1), 122–133. http://doi.org/10.4103/0973-1229.91587

MacIntyre, Alasdair. (2011). Utilitarianism and cost-benefit analyses: An essay on the relevance of moral philosophy to bureaucratic theory. In John Martin Gilroy and Murice L. Wade (eds.), *The moral dimensions of public policy choice: Beyond the market paradigm*. Pittsburgh, PA: University of Pittsburgh Press.

Merleau-Ponty, Maurice. (2004). *The world of perception, Causeries 1948*. London: Routledge.

Mill, J. S. (1991). Utilitarianism In J. Gray (Ed.), *On liberty and other essays*. Oxford: Oxford University Press.

Mitchell, M. (2019). *Artificial intelligence: A guide for thinking humans*. New York, NY: Farrar, Strauss and Giroux.

Nordgreen, T., Standal, B., Mannes, H., Haug, T., Sivertsen, B., Carlbring, P., … Havik, O. E. (2010). Guided self-help via internet for panic disorder: Dissemination across countries. *Computers in Human Behavior*, *26*(4), 592–596. http://doi.org/10.1016/j.chb.2009.12.011

Plato. (1993). *The Republic*. New York, NY: Oxford University Press.

Polsky, D., & Glick, H. (2009). Costing and cost analysis in randomized controlled trials: Caveat emptor. *PharmacoEconomics*, *27*(3), 179–188. http://doi.org/10.2165/00019053-200927030-00001

Popper, K. (1963). *Conjectures and refutations: The growth of scientific knowledge*. London: Routledge.

Popper, K. (2014). *The logic of scientific discovery*. Mansfield Centre, CT: Martino Publishing.

Seekles, W., van Straten, A., Beekman, A., van Marwijk, H., & Cuijpers, P. (2011). Effectiveness of guided self-help for depression and anxiety disorders in primary care: A pragmatic randomized controlled trial. *Psychiatry Research*, *187*(1–2), 113–120. http://doi.org/10.1016/j.psychres.2010.11.015

Sen, A. K. (2000). The discipline of cost-benefit analysis. *Journal of Legal Studies*, *29*(S2), 931–952. http://doi.org/10.1086/468100

Shepperd, J., Malone, W., & Sweeny, K. (2008). Exploring causes of the self-serving bias. *Social and Personality Psychology Compass*, *2*(2), 895–908. http://doi.org/10.1111/j.1751-9004.2008.00078.x

Smart, J. C. C. (1973). An outline of a system of utilitarian ethics. In J. C. C. Smart & B. Williams (Eds.), *Utilitarianism: For & against*. New York, NY: Cambridge University Press.

Snow, C. P. (1993). *The two cultures*. Cambridge: Cambridge University Press.

Stott, R., Wild, J., Grey, N., Liness, S., Warnock-Parkes, E., Commins, S., … Clark, D. M. (2013). Internet-delivered cognitive therapy for social anxiety disorder: A development pilot series. *Behavioural and Cognitive Psychotherapy*, *41*(4), 383–397. http://doi.org/10.1017/S1352465813000404

Walfish, S., McAlister, B., O'Donnell, P., & Lambert, M. J. (2012). An investigation of self-assessment bias in mental health providers. *Psychological Reports*, *110*(2), 639–644. http://doi.org/10.2466/02.07.17.Pr0.110.2.639-644

Watanabe, Tsuneo. (2010). Metascientific foundations for pluralism in psychology. *New Ideas in Psychology*, *28*(2), 253–262.

Weizenbaum, J. (1966). ELIZA: A computer program for the study of natural language communication between man and machine. *Communications of the ACM*, *9*(1), 36–45. http://doi.org/10.1145/365153.365168

Williams, B. (1973). A critique of utilitarianism. In J. C. C. Smart & B. Williams (Eds.), *Utilitarianism: For & against*. New York, NY: Cambridge University Press.

Woolfolk, Robert L. (2015). *The value of psychotherapy: The talking cure in an age of clinical science*. New York, NY: The Guilford Press.

7 Evidence-based practice in psychology

A tripartite concept?

A main rationale for introducing evidence-based practice in psychology was to replace the one-sided focus on scientific findings in empirically validated treatments (Levant, 2004; Peterson, 2004). The same rationale motivated the revisions of evidence-based medicine. These revisions recognise the distance between scientific findings and complex practices. Science essentially creates simplified descriptions of reality. The benefit of scientific models is that they can examine aspects of complex phenomena under controlled conditions (particularly in experimental research). This reduction makes it possible to make some justified inferences about the objects of inquiry. Reduction is not a problem in itself, but science must be understood as a simplification. It is problematic when science colonialises non-scientific realms.

When evidence-based practice in psychology was launched, the ideal was a threefold principle. The definition of evidence-based practice in psychology is the 'integration of the best available research with clinical expertise in the context of patient characteristics, culture, and preferences' (Levant, 2005, p. 5). In other words, the three intended components were:

- Best available research
- Clinical expertise
- Patients' characteristics, culture, and preferences

There is, however, lack of conceptual consistency in the policy statement. More specifically, evidence-based practice in psychology is not a tripartite concept. In the policy statement, evidence-based practice in psychology consists of only a single component, namely 'best available research.' This means that 'clinical expertise,' and 'patient characteristics, culture, and preferences' are neglected in the policy statement (Berg, 2019).

To understand why evidence-based practice in psychology fails to fulfil the ambition of being a tripartite concept, a conceptual differentiation is necessary. On the one hand, 'clinical expertise' and 'patient characteristics, culture, and preferences' are scientific objects of inquiry. They are

DOI: 10.4324/9781003512141-7

examined empirically to test whether they affect psychotherapy process and outcome. Some examples of scientific questions are: 'Which therapeutical characteristics or skills correlate positively with good patient outcomes?' or 'To what degree is including patients' preferences important for psychotherapy efficacy?' These are legitimate scientific questions. Studies have shown that common factors are significant in psychotherapy process and outcome (Lambert & Barley, 2002; Norcross & Lambert, 2011; Safran & Kraus, 2014; Safran & Muran, 2000; Wampold, 2001). Hence, the point is not that such research is futile. Nonetheless, the authors of the policy statement seem to have conflated some very significant conceptual distinctions. The individual clinical expertise of the therapist and the individual characteristics, culture/cultures, and preference of the patient are left out. Scientific theories normally compare 'clinical expertise' and 'patient characteristics, culture, and preferences' across individual cases. In contrast, the individual clinical expert and the individual patient are individual and unique. Research on clinical expertise is not the same as a practising individual clinical expert. Neither are the research on patient characteristics, culture, and preferences and an individual patient's characteristics, culture(s), and preferences identical. Hence, both clinical expertise and patient characteristics, culture, and preferences are scientific subcategories. In effect, evidence-based practice in psychology is not a threefold concept, but a concept consisting solely of 'best available research.'

Clinical expertise in the policy statement

The central rationale for the development of evidence-based medicine was criticism posed against expert-based medicine. Clinical experts' decisions have been shown to be biased. This fact makes the clinical expert an unreliable source of knowledge and action (Cochrane, 1999; Lilienfeld, Ritschel, Lynn, Cautin, & Latzman, 2013; The Evidence-Based Medicine Working Group, 1992). These fallacies and biases have been described in cognitive psychology and decision-making psychology. These biases involve anything from an incorrect understanding of quantitative metrics (Gigerenzer, 2003) to an overestimation of one's own skills and achievements (Lilienfeld et al., 2013; Shepperd, Malone, & Sweeny, 2008). Such biases, moreover, have informed the description of clinical expertise in the policy statement:

> Integral to clinical expertise is an awareness of the limits of one's knowledge and skills and attention to the heuristics and biases— both cognitive and affective—that can affect clinical judgment.
>
> (American Psychological Association, 2006, p. 276)

In the quote, the research literature defines the limits of expert knowledge. The research literature, moreover, describes the different 'heuristics and biases' that may affect clinical decision-making. Being an expert is, in other words, a matter of knowing 'best available research evidence.'

The expert is modelled on a scientist: '[...] clinical expertise [...] frame and test hypotheses and interventions in practice' like a 'local clinical scientist' (American Psychological Association, 2006, p. 275–276). Because hypotheses testing has been a success in science, it is assumed that the same mode will guide the clinical expert towards good decision-making. When hypotheses testing works optimally, its most prominent features are being critical and tentative. Yet, the formulation of accurate hypotheses is a meticulous effort which normally results in specific predictions about a delimited and relatively stable (or at least stabilised) object of inquiry. This is not a good depiction of the more dynamic form of clinical interaction. The patient's problems are rarely as delimited as object of inquiry in scientific studies. Although, naturally, the hypotheses in question are clinical hypotheses, the expert is nonetheless modelled on a scientist.

The policy statement refers to empirical literature suggesting that the clinical expert has a greater impact on the outcome than specific treatment methods. Specific treatment methods refer to the interventions from a psychotherapy school. Levant (2005) notes that: 'In psychotherapy, for example, individual therapist effects (within treatments) account for 5 to 8% of the outcome variance' (p. 277). Furthermore, a distinction runs between research on specific interventions and research on a specific application of different interventions: 'Research suggests that sensitivity and flexibility in administering therapeutic interventions produces better outcomes than rigid application of manuals or principles' (Levant, 2005, p. 278). This provides an empirical base for delivering therapeutic interventions with some flexibility as opposed to the rigid application of manuals. This justification is, however, based on the component 'best available research.' This illustrates how the current description of 'clinical expertise' is a mere subcategory of the component 'best available research.' Therefore, we should provide arguments in favour of including the individual clinical expert in a regulatory principle.

Individual clinical expertise

Wieten (2018) has described three different conceptualisations of clinical expertise within evidence-based medicine (relevant to evidence-based practice in psychology). The first tradition stems from decision-making psychology, which focuses on how clinical experts often make poor decisions (Kahneman & Klein, 2009; Lilienfeld, McKay, & Hollon, 2018; Lilienfeld et al., 2013). This tradition largely reflects the scepticism towards clinical experts in Cochrane (1999) and, to a certain degree, in empirically validated treatment forms. As noted, this conceptualisation of 'clinical expertise' plays a major part in evidence-based practice in psychology (Levant, 2005).

Other traditions, however, have a more positive take on expertise. Their conceptualisations are not directly tied to scientific findings. One of these is (Dreyfus & Dreyfus, 1980) phenomenological model of expertise. Phenomenologist Martin Heidegger (1953) was probably the most important inspiration for Dreyfus and Dreyfus' expert model. He wrote about the relationship between the Greek word *techne* and expertise. *Techne* provides the prefix in the word technology. The delimiting understanding of *techne* implies an instrumentalism; *techne* is normally understood as knowledge and skills about how means realise predefined ends. Heidegger (1953), however, argued that this understanding leaves out an important aspect of this term. *Techne* involves a deeply ingrained expertise. The expert's actions spring from a context (i.e., society and culture), which must inform our understanding of the action. This means that realising a given aim implies that one is 'already' within a context where certain aims are considered good and others bad (Heidegger, 1953). According to Tjeltveit (1999), social and cultural moral standards affect what is considered good aims in psychotherapy. The aims for psychotherapy are, in other words, culturally contingent and predicated on values. Both the means we use and the aims we establish must be considered in the light of this fact (Tjeltveit, 1999, 2004).

Dreyfus and Dreyfus (1980) model of expertise describes how novices and experts solve tasks differently. Compared to experts, novices are more rulebound and have more fragmented problem-solving strategies. Moreover, novices are more self-observing and unable to relate their performance to the situation holistically. Conversely, experts have a more holistic understanding of the situation, and they adapt their performance relatively flexibly. This involves handling unforeseen situations appropriately. Experts are absorbed in the activity and perform in more intuitive ways. Hence, the clinical expert does not correspond each independent clinical action to the research literature, although the professional perspective and practice may be anchored in scientific knowledge. According to Dreyfus and Dreyfus' (1980) model, the expert transcends science but that does not entail necessarily diverging from science.

The third tradition is Science and Technology Studies (STS) (Wieten, 2018). Science and Technology Studies analyses the complex mutual interplay between society, science, technology, and policy (Jasanoff, 2016). Collins and Evans (2007) have explored questions connected to expertise within Science and Technology Studies. Collins and Evans' (2007) taxonomy challenges that science is the only valid source of knowledge. However, it is not anti-science. The primary intention is to go beyond the descriptions offered by science. Collins and Evans (2007) have provided an extensive taxonomy of expertise. Here, we will only focus on three forms of expertise: contributory expertise, interactional expertise, and ubiquitous expertise. In their general account of the development within the understanding of expertise, Collins and Evans (2007) wrote:

> Over the last half-century, the most important transformation in the way expertise has been understood is a move away from seeing knowledge and ability as quasi logical or mathematical and toward a more wisdom-based or competence-based model.
>
> (p. 23)

What kinds of expertise is it, then, that goes beyond scientific models holding relevance for psychotherapy? Collins and Evans' (2007) taxonomy is influenced by phenomenological thinking (like that of Dreyfus and Dreyfus (1980)). Collins and Evans (2007) coin the kind of knowledge depicted in Dreyfus and Dreyfus (1980) as 'contributory expertise.' The name reflects that this kind of expertise can only be acquired through direct contribution or participation. This is the expertise that the psychotherapist acquires through clinical practice.

'Interactional expertise' is the type of expertise acquired through interacting with experts without having direct practical experience. Interactional expertise provides the ability to understand what a group of experts are talking about, without possessing the same knowledge or skills oneself. An example of a relevant form of interactional expertise is understanding other relevant professionals.

'Ubiquitous expertise' is the general and extensive expertise needed to live in a human society. The most obvious examples are linguistic competence and moral sensibility. These examples illustrate that ubiquitous expertise is a precondition for being able to work as a clinical psychologist. An important point here is, of course, the difference between 'best available research' and ubiquitous expertise. This takes us back to Smith and Pell's (2003) article where they (ironically) wanted to test whether a parachute was an effective mean to handle 'gravitational challenges.' Many actions are not based on science. Some examples could be 'the pace of walking,' 'the firmness and duration of a handshake,' or 'how to sneeze politely.' These, and thousands of other actions, are performed by virtue of understanding the codes of a culture and/or an individual.

The three kinds of expertise in Collins and Evans (2007) illustrate how experts transcend scientific claims about what it is that constitute good psychotherapeutic practice. Therefore, they contribute to an understanding of why it is necessary to include this dimension in a regulatory principle for psychotherapy practice.

Patient characteristics, culture, and preferences in the policy statement

It is useful to divide 'patient characteristics, culture, and preferences' into two new subcategories. One aspect of this component is patient characteristics that are significant for treatment. Cultural background is an example of such characteristics, but we might also have mentioned other characteristics such as gender, sexual orientation, political ideals, or age. This subcategory, which provides several parameters for assessing what kind of person the patient is, may enable the therapist to be more nuanced.

The other aspect of this component is what the patients prefer. Two patients with equal characteristics (equal cultural background, gender, age, sexual orientation, etc.) may have (widely) different preferences. The 'preference' in 'patient characteristics, culture, and preferences' is particularly important because it signals the patient's rights to influence her or his treatment. We might let patient characteristics (such as cultural background) inform treatment through scientific findings. This, however, is not possible when it comes to the patient's individual preferences, simply because they are individual. We may illustrate this point by two very brief examples. Picture two patients with different characteristics. One is a woman born in North Africa. She is 81 years old and visually impaired. She enjoys listening to classical music and visiting or being visited by her family. The other is a man who is a third-generation immigrant from South-East Asia. He is 19 years old, lives with his parents, and enjoys playing video games. Let us say that these two, even after being informed about the differences connected to their treatments, had identical preferences. Should the therapist treat them differently? Empirical analyses may indicate that it would be appropriate to treat them differently. The clinical expert might also have clinical experiences that indicate that these patients with their differing backgrounds and life situations should receive different treatments. It is, however, difficult to defend different treatments based on the final component (i.e., 'patient characteristics, culture, and preferences'). The most important for introducing this component was to secure the patient's rights to influence their treatment. It would, thus, be ethically problematic to argue that the patient's individual characteristics should trump the patient's individual preferences in clinical decision-making.

In the policy statement, the component 'patient characteristics, culture, and preferences' is justified as follows:

> Normative data on "what works for whom" (…) provide essential guides to effective practice. Nevertheless, psychological services are most likely to be effective when responsive to the patient's specific problems, strengths, personality, sociocultural context, and preferences.
>
> (Levant, 2005, p. 278)

The justification for including 'patient characteristics, culture, and preferences' is that science shows it will result in a more 'effective practice.' This means that the most important ethical justification for including patient preferences is left out of the policy statement.

Individual patient preferences

Patients normally have extensive ethical and legal rights to influencing their own treatment. Patient's vision of a good life may vary considerably. Thus, patient preferences need to be a part of (good) treatment. At the same time, there is an important distinction between patient preferences and autonomy. Patient preferences denote what the patient wants without requirements concerning *how* the patient justifies their aims. Patient autonomy, in contrast, denotes informed and independent decisions. Pellegrino and Thomasma (1993) argued that autonomy entails freedom from the interference from third parties and insufficient understanding. This means that patient preferences do not imply patient autonomy. The patient should have relevant information about the benefits and disadvantages as well as the aims of the different treatment forms. Furthermore, it is crucial that patients are allowed to choose without being steered towards a given course of action (by the therapist or significant others).

The distinction between patient preferences and patient autonomy requires some nuance. As patient autonomy implies certain freedoms, autonomy may only be achieved when integrating patient preferences with the remaining components. The patient may be considered autonomous only when the patient is adequately informed about 'best available research' and when the decision is not dictated to others. This means that the shift from patient preferences to patient autonomy requires integration (which will be the main topic of Chapter 8).

Fulford (2008, 2011, 2013) has introduced an approach called value-based practice. It aims to facilitate patient autonomy in mental healthcare. Value-based practice intends to supplement evidence-based practice; scientific facts are integrated with the patient's values. Integration is achieved as therapists acquire the skills to identify the values of psychotherapy and integrate them in clinical practice. On the one hand, value-based practice improves evidence-based practice in psychology because values are integrated to clinical practice. On the other hand, it fails to acknowledge the extent to which psychotherapy is imbued with values. One example of a dimension which is not acknowledged is the 'ethos' of psychotherapy. In value-based practice, the scientific evidence on whether a given approach has a given effect is presented as a 'fact.' However, patient autonomy also includes freedom from lapses in knowledge. Hence, an autonomous patient is also familiar with the aims of treatment (e.g., the ethos of different psychotherapy schools). Consequently, it is ethically imperative to have an adequate conceptualisation of psychotherapy – also with regards to patient autonomy.

Integration in evidence-based practice in psychology

So far, we have seen that the policy statement for evidence-based practice in psychology is not a threefold model. The current version conflates (1) clinical expertise and patient characteristics, culture, and preferences as scientific research objects and (2) the individual clinical expertise and individual (characteristics, culture, and) preferences. The first objective of this chapter was to try to introduce this distinction. The next step is to try to outline how the different components should relate to one another.

The relationship between the components of evidence-based practice in psychology may be interpreted in different ways. We may consider alternatives where one of the components should hold precedence. In evidence-based practice in psychology, the most likely candidate is 'best available research.' Norcross, Hogan, and Koocher (2008) claimed that: '[…] not all three pillars are equal. Research assumes priority in [evidence-based practice]' (p. 5). The quote from Norcross et al. (2008) has severe repercussions for psychotherapy. It is empirical knowledge about (means) effectiveness that should guide psychotherapy. Treatment should only be adjusted in accordance with the clinical expert and the patient's preferences.

Another way of conceptualising the three components is that they should have equal impact. It is, as it were, difficult to formalise an unequivocal understanding of 'equal' in this context. We may imagine two different clinical scenarios. In one scenario, the research results are relatively clear, the clinician prefers a treatment that corresponds to the research results, and the patient does not have any specific preferences. We may, however, also consider quite a different scenario. Here, the research evidence is ambiguous, the clinician's expertise diverges with the research evidence, and where the patient has clear (diverging) preferences. 'Equality' would have different meanings in the two scenarios. Notwithstanding, it is integration that makes practice 'evidence-based.' Hence, it is a necessary feature. At a minimum, the three components should be considered and play a role in practice.

However, it is worth asking why we should have three, rather than one single component. Referring to developments in medicine without justification rests on a (weak) authority argument. In the following, I will outline how we may justify the three components in evidence-based practice in psychology.

The separation of powers

One way of approaching the relationship between the different components is to see them as expressions of different interests of power. Winter (2016) defines power as 'the ability or capacity to produce intended effects' (p. 160). The connection between a regulatory principle and power is quite obvious. First, it is a matter of establishing legitimacy for a profession among other professions, authorities, users, and so on. Furthermore, it has the purpose of bringing about certain effects. The effects sought in evidence-based practice in psychology is indicated by its three components. At the same time, evidence-based practice in psychology is defined as the integration of its three components. Hence, there is a tension between the different power interests that constitute the three parts and the aim to integrate them.

A considerable literature connects scientific knowledge to power interest. These interests may simply entail an 'interest' in finding out 'how the world is.' This knowledge, in turn, provides an opportunity to steer the world in an intended direction. If we know the causes of good mental health, we also know the means to provide it (Habermas, 1972). Other analyses have, however, revealed more intricate relationships between power and knowledge. In such analyses, power works subconsciously to shape the premises for scientific knowledge (Foucault, 1977; Nietzsche, 1968). Power factors play a part in issues connected to the expert's authority and in providing the patient with the power to shape healthcare services (Elwyn et al., 2012; Veatch, 2009).

As the three different power interests of the three components of evidence-based practice in psychology do not necessarily coincide, conflicts of interest will (probably) arise. D.G. Winter (2016) has, however, argued that the taming of power is often desirable when different powers collide:

> Power is a necessary dimension of all human enterprises. It can inspire and illuminate, but it can also corrupt, oppress, and destroy. Therefore, taming power has been a central moral and political question for most of human history. Writers, theorists, and researchers have suggested many methods and mechanisms for taming power [...] [such as] separation of powers.
>
> (p. 160)

As power is a necessary aspect of life, the challenge is to tame power to ensure a constructive use of power. In this context, this means that the three components are integrated in constructive ways.

In political theory, principles have been developed for preventing concentration of power (Winther (2016), on his part, envisions other solutions).

It is presumed that separation of power may have a corrective effect on the execution of power and that different institutions of power may adjust each other in appropriate ways. In political philosophy, Charles Montesquieu (1689–1755) is known for having created a political system that separates between executive, legislative, and judiciary power (Krause, 2000). We may conceive of a related justification for having three different components of evidence-based practice in psychology. The three components may have a corrective effect on each other and may compensate for the destructive potential that is latent in each component. Herein also lies a central justification for integrating the three components: The three components of evidence-based practice in psychology prevent bias and inappropriate concentration of power interests.

Ideal types of healthcare systems

To clarify the problematic aspects of the three components, we may imagine how a healthcare system where one of the three components worked unrestrictedly would have looked like. These hypothetical models are ideal types (and do not reflect any existing healthcare systems). The concept of ideal types originates from Max Weber. He used the concept to describe the typical features of different phenomena. Ideal types do not provide exhaustive descriptions of actual existing phenomena (Weber, 2011). In this context, they help us highlight the problems tied to the three components. This, in turn, legitimise a tripartite regulatory principle, despite the hypothetical nature of the ideal types.

To outline a regulatory principle informed by scientific findings, we must first give a succinct account of science. In a science like psychology, the definition of science varies (Watanabe, 2010). Narrow definitions normally delimit science to natural sciences. In contrast, a broader definition includes social sciences and humanities. As already noted, randomised controlled trials are deemed superior to other methods in evidence-based practice in psychology. Randomised controlled trials aim to disclose causal relationships between variables (based on a given conceptualisation of causality) (Anjum, 2016; Anjum & Mumford, 2016). In psychotherapy research, this typically means to correlate variables with outcomes (in temporal succession and with experimental control). In addition, randomised controlled trials may be used to estimate the cost of different kinds of treatment (Polsky & Glick, 2009). A healthcare system based solely on randomised controlled trials would be rigidly bureaucratic. In a bureaucratic healthcare service, scientific findings would determine what treatments that would be offered to patient groups. Individual differences, beyond those categorising patients in research, would be deemed irrelevant. Neither patient's preferences nor the clinical expert's translation of scientific findings would be relevant. The clinical interaction would, in other words, be dictated by scientific findings. This ideal was, however, abandoned in the ideal undergirding evidence-based practice in psychology (Levant, 2004; Peterson, 2004).

We may also imagine a system dominated by the clinical expert. We can characterise such a system as paternalistic. Paternalistic thinking has greatly impacted our understanding of different professions, not the least medicine (Timmermans & Berg, 2003). In paternalistic systems, the expert acts on behalf of lay people. It is based on the presumption that the expert is better informed about a given problem. Thus, it is presumably in the best interests of patients that the expert acts on their behalf. In a paternalistic system, the expert dictates and the patient receives the treatment. Although the expert has undergone training, the choices are not necessarily founded upon scientific knowledge. As noted, paternalistic medicine was critiqued on this very basis. The expert presumably possesses some general skills that enables good clinical decision-making. In a strictly paternalistic system, the patient's right to participate is very limited. Considerations such as the patient's preferences and values are, in other words, not relevant for the treatment.

Finally, we may imagine an ideal typical system dominated by the patient. We can call it a consumerist system. In the consumerist system, the patient's preferences determine the form of treatment. The clinical expert simply facilitates and is not a critical partner. Scientific findings connected to the effects of different treatment alternatives are only relevant to the extent that the patient wants them to be. The patient's preferences and values should be a part of psychotherapy. Yet, if they were to work unrestrictedly, a range of problems would arise. In some cases, this would be evident. We can imagine an extreme hypothetical situation where the patient is a sadist. He or she seeks help to perfect subjecting others to psychological discomfort. We may also imagine a patient who desires a kind of treatment that would obviously harm the patient in question. In such cases, ethical considerations would outweigh the patient's preferences.

In *The Ethics of Authenticity*, Taylor (1991) argued that a style of reasoning has emerged in Western societies. The individual rights that originated in the Enlightenment Era have become reduced to a remnant where individual's wishes and desires are considered the only valid ethical justification for actions. However, according to Taylor (1991), all understanding emerges within a social and historical context which must be incorporated in ethical assessments. There is a difficult balance to strike regarding the patient's right to participate in decision-making. Nonetheless, one should problematise the challenges connected to a scenario where the patient's preferences are allowed to work unrestrictedly. A professional service entails some duties with regard to effects of that service, both ethically and legally.

Scientific findings are made relevant to a clinical context by a clinical expert and through the preferences of a specific patient. If this does not occur, scientific research may become the tyrant that Sackett (1997) warned against. Clinical expertise is refined by scientific findings and by the patient's preferences. Without scientific findings, there is a risk that experts will make suboptimal decisions. Without including the patient's preferences, a decision may be both scientifically informed and in accordance with clinical expertise, yet unable to help an individual patient with his or her individual needs. At the same time, scientific findings may contribute to clarifying the outcomes that are likely to spring from different treatment alternatives. Thus, scientific findings are important in the creation of autonomous patients. As the three components work correctively against each other, it becomes possible to deliberate on the most relevant considerations for making good clinical decisions. First, this demonstrates that we need three components. Second, it shows that they need to be integrated. It is through integration of the different powers that the different components become adjusted and may work to benefit individual patients.

Conclusion

There are many reasons why the current formulation of evidence-based practice in psychology should be discarded. A policy statement which is not conceptually consistent can hardly claim legitimacy. There are two alternatives. In one of them, evidence-based practice would be defined as a model consisting of a singular component. This is how the Canadian Psychological Association (2012) defines evidence-based practice in psychology. The benefit of such a model is its parsimony. The other alternative is to reformulate evidence-based practice in psychology to actually compound three distinct components. As best available research is insufficient to regulate psychotherapy, evidence-based practice in psychology should encompass more than this component. A clinical expert is necessary to assess scientific findings and translate them to clinical practice. It is also crucial to incorporate the patient's preferences and to strive for patient autonomy. Although it is demanding to integrate these three elements, it is important to achieve good clinical practice. Furthermore, seeing the three different components as powers will make the benefits visible of integrating them (as well as the disadvantages of letting each component work unrestrictedly).

References

American Psychological Association. (2006). Policy statement on evidence-based practice in psychology. *American Psychologist*, *61*(4), 271–285. https://doi.org/10.1037/0003-066X.61.4.271

Anjum, R. L. (2016). Evidence Based or Person Centered: An ontological debate. *European Journal for Person Centered Healthcare*, *4*(2), 421–429. http://doi.org/10.5750/ejpch.v4i2.1152

Anjum, R. L., & Mumford, S. D. (2016). A philosophical argument against evidence-based policy. *Journal of Evaluation in Clinical Practice*, 1045–1050. http://doi.org/10.1111/jep.12578

Berg, H. (2019). Evidence-based practice in psychology fails to be tripartite: A conceptual critique of the scientocentrism in evidence-based practice in psychology. *Frontiers in Psychology*, *10*, 2253. http://doi.org/10.3389/fpsyg.2019.02253

Canadian Psychological Association. (2012). *Evidence-Based Practice of Psychological Treatments: A Canadian Perspective*. Retrieved from https://cpa.ca/docs/File/Practice/Report_of_the_EBP_Task_Force_FINAL_Board_Approved_2012.pdf

Cochrane, A. L. (1999). *Effectiveness and efficiency: Random reflections on health services*. London: Royal Society of Medicine Press.

Collins, H., & Evans, R. (2007). *Rethinking expertise*. Chicago, IL: The University of Chicago Press.

Dreyfus, S. E., & Dreyfus, H. L. (1980). *A five-stage model of the mental activities involved in directed skill acquisition*. Berkely, CA: California University Berkeley Operations Research Center.

Elwyn, G., Frosch, D., Thomson, R., Joseph-Williams, N., Lloyd, A., Kinnersley, P., … Barry, M. (2012). Shared decision making: A model for clinical practice. *Journal of General Internal Medicine*, *27*(10), 1361–1367. http://doi.org/10.1007/s11606-012-2077-6

Foucault, M. (1977). *Discipline and punish: The birth of the prison*. London: Allen Lane.

Fulford, K. W. M. (2008). Values-based practice: A new partner to evidence-based practice and a first for psychiatry? *Mens Sana Monographs*, *6*(1), 10–21. http://doi.org/10.4103/0973-1229.40565

Fulford, K. W. M. (2011). The value of evidence and evidence of values: Bringing together values-based and evidence-based practice in policy and service development in mental health. *Journal of Evaluation in Clinical Practice*, *17*(5), 976–987.

Fulford, K. W. M. (2013). Values-based practice: Fulford's dangerous idea. *Journal of Evaluation in Clinical Practice*, *19*(3), 537–546. http://doi.org/10.1111/jep.12054

Gigerenzer, G. (2003). *Reckoning with risk: Learning to live with uncertainty*. London: Penguin Books.

Habermas, J. (1972). *Knowledge and human interests*. London: Heinemann.

Heidegger, M. (1953). The question concerning technology. In D. F. Krell (Ed.), *Heidegger: Basic writings*. London: Routledge.

Jasanoff, S. (2016). *The ethics of invention: Technology and the human future*. New York, NY: W. W. Norton & Company.

Kahneman, D., & Klein, G. (2009). Conditions for intuitive expertise: A failure to disagree. *American Psychologist*, *64*(6), 515–526. http://doi.org/10.1037/a0016755

Krause, S. (2000). The Spirit of Separate Powers in Montesquieu. *The Review of Politics*, *62*(2), 231–265. http://doi.org/10.1017/S0034670500029454

Lambert, M. J., & Barley, D. E. (2002). Psychotherapy relationships that work: Evidence-based responsiveness. In J. C. Norcross (Ed.), *Psychotherapy relationships that work* (pp. 17–32). New York, NY: Oxford University Press.

Levant, Ronald F. (2005). *Report of the 2005 Presidential Task Force on evidence-based practice*. American Psychological Association.

Lilienfeld, S. O., McKay, D., & Hollon, S. D. (2018). Why randomised controlled trials of psychological treatments are still essential. *The Lancet Psychiatry*, *5*(7), 536–538. http://doi.org/10.1016/S2215-0366(18)30045-2

Lilienfeld, S. O., Ritschel, L. A., Lynn, S. J., Cautin, R. L., & Latzman, R. D. (2013). Why many clinical psychologists are resistant to evidence-based practice: Root causes and constructive remedies. *Clinical Psychology Review*, *33*(7), 883–900. http://doi.org/10.1016/j.cpr.2012.09.008

Nietzsche, F. (1968). *The will to power*. New York, NY: Vintage Books.

Norcross, J. C., Hogan, T. P., & Koocher, G. P. (2008). *Clinician's guide to evidence based practices: Mental health and the addictions*. New York, NY: Oxford University Press.

Norcross, J. C., & Lambert, M. J. (2011). Evidence-based therapy relationships. In J. C. Norcross (Ed.), *Psychotherapy relationships that work: Evidence-based responsiveness* (2nd ed., pp. 3–24). New York, NY: Oxford University Press.

Pellegrino, E. D., & Thomasma, D. C. (1993). *The virtues in medical practice*. New York, NY: Oxford University Press.

Peterson, D. R. (2004). Science, scientism, and professional responsibility. *Clinical Psychology: Science and Practice*, 11(2), 196–210. https://doi.org/10.1093/clipsy.bph072

Polsky, D., & Glick, H. (2009). Costing and cost analysis in randomized controlled trials: Caveat emptor. *PharmacoEconomics*, *27*(3), 179–188. http://doi.org/10.2165/00019053-200927030-00001

Sackett, D. L. (1997). Evidence-based medicine. *Seminars in Perinatology*, *21*(1), 3–5. https://doi.org/10.1016/S0146-0005(97)80013-4

Safran, J. D., & Kraus, J. (2014). Alliance ruptures, impasses, and enactments: A relational perspective. *Psychotherapy*, *51*(3), 381–387. http://doi.org/10.1037/a0036815

Safran, J. D., & Muran, J. C. (2000). *Negotiating the therapeutic alliance*. New York, NY: The Guilford Press.

Shepperd, J., Malone, W., & Sweeny, K. (2008). Exploring causes of the self-serving bias. *Social and Personality Psychology Compass*, *2*(2), 895–908. http://doi.org/10.1111/j.1751-9004.2008.00078.x

Smith, Gordon C. S., & Pell, Jill P. (2003). Parachute use to prevent death and major trauma related to gravitational challenge: Systematic review of randomised controlled trials. *British Medical Journal*, *327*, 1459–1461. https://doi.org/10.1136/bmj.327.7429.1459

Taylor, C. (1991). *The ethics of authenticity*. Cambridge, MA: Harvard University Press.

The Evidence-Based Medicine Working Group. (1992). Evidence-based medicine: A new approach to teaching the practice of medicine. *JAMA*, *268*(17), 2420–2425. http://doi.org/10.1001/jama.1992.03490170092032

Timmermans, Stefan, and Berg, Marc (2003). *The gold standard: The challenge of evidence-based medicine and standardization in health care*. Philadelphia, PA: Temple University Press.

Tjeltveit, Alan C. (1999). *Ethics and values in psychotherapy*. London: Routledge.

Veatch, R. M. (2009). *Patient, heal thyself: How the new medicine puts the patient in charge*. New York, NY: Oxford University Press.

Wampold, B. (2001). *The great psychotherapy debate: Models, methods, and findings*. Mahwah, NJ: Lawrence Erlbaum Associates.

Watanabe, T. (2010). Metascientific foundations for pluralism in psychology. *New Ideas in Psychology*, *28*(2), 253–262. http://doi.org/10.1016/j.newideapsych.2009.09.019

Weber, M. (2011). *Methodology of the social sciences*. New Brunswick, NJ: Transaction Publishers.

Wieten, S. (2018). Expertise in evidence-based medicine: A tale of three models. *Philosophy, Ethics, and Humanities in Medicine 13*(1), 2–2. http://doi.org/10.1186/s13010-018-0055-2

Winter, D. G. (2016). Taming power: Generative historical consciousness. *American Psychologist*, *71*(3), 160–174. http://doi.org/10.1037/a0039312

8 Clinical expertise as therapeutic virtues

The previous chapter had two main purposes. The first was to show that the current version of evidence-based practice in psychology does not have three components. In the policy statement, 'clinical expertise' and 'patients' characteristics, culture, and preferences' are defined as scientific subcategories. The second purpose was to provide a justification for why the policy statement should contain three components. A principle of regulation that consists of a single component is unsuited to regulate a complex practice like psychotherapy.

In this chapter, the aim is to take a closer look at how the three components may be integrated. Integration has been subject to little discussion in the literature on evidence-based practice in psychology (Norcross et al., 2008). This absence is remarkable in and by itself. There may be significant gaps between 'best available research evidence,' 'clinical expertise,' and 'patients' characteristics, culture, and preferences.' This means that the integration of the three components can be demanding. That, in turn, would presumably result in a need to discuss integration.

As noted, the historical backdrop of evidence-based practice in psychology reflected a belief in the utility of science and a distrust in experts. Although this distrust has been excessive at times, there is still something to be learned from this history. Several of the empirical studies conducted in the wake of Cochrane (1999) illustrate how important science can be in healthcare practices (Timmermans og Berg, 2003). Notwithstanding, there are genuine challenges connected to scientific practices failing to live up to acceptable standards. Two examples are publication bias and p-hacking (Gupta, 2014; Hengartner, 2018). Such practices clearly compromise the practical utility of research. Science, moreover, cannot function as an unequivocal corrective to clinical expertise. This point is reflected in the fact that science consists of simplified descriptions of complex phenomena. Thus, science must be adapted (or translated) to be useful in the practical sphere.

Integration means to bring together or combine things with one another and form a unit (or to reassemble something into an original whole).

DOI: 10.4324/9781003512141-8

The unit or whole is the therapeutic intervention (in a broad sense). Integration of 'the best available research with clinical expertise in the context of patient characteristics, culture, and preferences' (Levant, 2005, p. 5) means to unite the three components in an intervention (or alternatively in a series of different interventions).

In a clinical context, the clinical expert is responsible for integrating the three components in evidence-based practice in psychology. The clinical expert must know the 'best available research evidence.' Furthermore, this knowledge must be adapted to fit the individual 'patient's characteristics, culture, and preferences.' In addition, the clinical expert ought to be aware of their own impact in clinical practice. Norcross et al. (2008) have claimed that the clinical expert holds a central role in evidence-based practice in psychology. Yet, Norcross et al. (2008) noted that the clinical expert and clinical integration have not been subject to extensive analysis.

Psychotherapy normally aims at realising a better life for the patient and, thus, normative ideals are constitutive for psychotherapy. As we have seen, normative ethics are theories defining goodness and/or rightness. This means that the normative ideals of psychotherapy practice are inextricably connected to normative ethics. When we designate a treatment as 'good,' we use a benchmark from normative ethics which provides the criteria for assessing 'goodness.' This is reflected in the 'ethos' of psychotherapy (described in Chapter 5).

Virtue ethics

Virtue ethics defines 'the good' based on the source of the action. In clinical practice, the source of integration is the clinical expert. The context-dependent purpose to be realised is a better life for the patient. The patient is a 'context dependent purpose' in the sense that each patient differs in clinically relevant ways. Patients are normally quite active contributors in psychotherapy. While the patient has extensive rights, the patient carries little (if any) responsibility for the quality of the treatment. It is, moreover, the responsibility of the clinical expert to integrate the patient's preferences. Of course, the patients' preferences must be conveyed by the patients themselves. Yet, it is the clinical expert that is the integrator. Note that this does not say anything about whether the patient is active in treatment or not. The point here is the act of integration.

A virtue is a stable character trait and motivation. Virtues enable a person to achieve a given goal (more often than not). The goal, however, may vary considerably. Kindness is a virtue which allows us to establish and maintain good relations, and perhaps also a good self-image. 'Moderation' allows us to balance pleasure and duty in a good way. In short, there are a range of virtues that are necessary to living a good life.

Many virtue ethicists maintain that the highest end for a person is *eudaimonia*. *Eudaimonia* is normally translated into happiness, but flourishing is probably a better word. While happiness is often associated with certain emotions, *eudaimonia* designates how people function when they function optimally (Waterman, 2008). This means that virtues are not only relevant for our understanding of clinical expertise but also for many of the changes that psychotherapy aims to bring about. Therapeutic virtues are those capacities that make the clinical expert capable of helping others to live a satisfactory life. While the goal of psychotherapy is typically (not exclusively) some lasting changes in the patient.

Zagzebski (1996) defines virtue as: 'a deep and enduring acquired excellence of a person, involving a characteristic motivation to produce a certain desired end and reliable success in bringing about that end' (p. 137). A central point in Zagzebski's (1996) definition is that it contains acquired skills. The development of different virtues demands cultivation. If we fail to develop virtues, we develop (more or less severe) character flaws or vices. In psychotherapy, we may think of vices as the therapist capacities that impedes good therapy. Waring (2016) has provided a more extensive definition of virtue as: '[A] multi-track character trait or disposition […] [that] involve a complex mindset of fine inner states that inform an array of emotional responses, desires, motivations, reasons, and values' (p. 59). According to this definition, virtues involve justifications, values, and skills that make it possible to realise a given goal. When persons possess relevant virtues, their emotions, values, justifications, motivation, and skills harmonise. Thus, the person wants and is able to achieve the relevant goals. For a psychotherapist, this would typically mean to help a patient to a better life. Another aspect of virtues is that these capacities are quite stable. It is not enough to have a high potential; one must have the capacities to act consistently. Therefore, the combination of skills and motivation is important. This explains why desire is a part of Waring's (2016) definition of virtue.

Some scholars have connected virtue ethics to evidence-based practice. Zarkovich and Upshur (2002) have re-interpreted evidence-based medicine using concepts from virtue ethics. Some definitions of evidence-based medicine rest upon specific virtues such as 'conscientiousness' and 'judiciousness' (Zarkovich og Upshur, 2002). Others have shown that virtue ethics is relevant to understand clinical expertise and integration in evidence-based practice in psychology. To be able to integrate, the clinical expert must possess certain capacities and skills. In virtue ethics, the Greek term *phronesis* or practical wisdom denotes this capacity. The clinical expert must also possess virtues that correspond to the three components of evidence-based practice in psychology: 'best available research evidence,' 'clinical expertise,' and 'patients' characteristics, culture, and preferences.' Hence, we can designate these virtues: epistemic virtues, self-reflexive virtues, and relational virtues (Berg, 2020). In this chapter, we will first take a closer look at practical wisdom. Next, we will consider the virtues that correspond to the three components of evidence-based practice in psychology (epistemic virtues, self-reflexive virtues, and relational virtues).

Practical wisdom

To understand practical wisdom, we should turn briefly to Ancient Greece where this concept originated. The concept originates from a discussion between Plato and Aristotle. According to Plato, abstract knowledge (e.g., what is justice) will lead to good acts (e.g., judiciousness). Aristotle only partly agrees with Plato. Good acts require more than abstract knowledge. To act in good ways, we need practical experience. The chief reason for this is that the right action must be contextualised. It is very difficult to understand the ethical matrices of concrete situations without some experience.

Aristotle (2009) presented a knowledge typology (as sketched in Chapter 6). He distinguished between three forms of knowledge: *episteme*, *techne*, and *phronesis*. *Episteme* is pure theoretical knowledge (non-applied knowledge). Examples are pure mathematics or theoretical philosophy. *Techne* refers to practical skills. Some examples are the skills for building a boat or to chop down a tree. *Phronesis* or practical wisdom, however, is distinct from both of these types of knowledge. While *episteme* is theoretical, necessarily true, knowledge, *phronesis* is a practical and a more approximate type of knowledge. Of course, according to the contemporary understanding, little empirical psychological knowledge is necessarily true. A more relevant distinction runs between robust empirical knowledge and the application of this knowledge in complex practices. Even robust scientific findings are reductive. They always differ from practical applications. Hence, the difference between scientific findings and the appropriate course of action in a practical situation is relevant. *Phronesis* helps us clarify this distinction.

Techne is knowledge and skills to achieve certain pre-established goals. *Phronesis*, in contrast, refers to the combined skill of assessing and achieving the good outcome in concrete situations (Aristotle, 2009). Highly standardised psychotherapy treatments are modelled on *techne*. In such treatments, both the purpose and the means are pre-established. In standardised psychotherapeutic practice, the goal is to emulate the steps that has been scientifically tested. Therefore, the psychotherapist should refrain from deviating from the treatment manuals. In structured treatments, the preferences of individual patients are less relevant. In less structured treatments, however, they are a natural part of the therapy. Precisely because it is concerned with realising context-specific goals, *phronesis* is relevant for individualised treatment. Individualisation is inherent to evidence-based practice in psychology (due to the component patient's preferences). In virtue ethics, *phronesis* functions as an overarching virtue. *Phronesis* coordinates the other moral virtues. Thus, an actor can make good individualised practical decisions. Radden and Sadler (2010) have provided a definition:

> [P}hronesis allows us to deliberate about things with ends or goals in mind, and to discern and enact right action. A grasp of particulars is required for phronesis, so it comprises cleverness (in the ability to find what is needed to achieve an end or goal), perception (in order to notice facts in a situation), and finally, understanding (noûs), a common and practical good sense.
>
> (pp. 144–145)

Phronesis is not a purely theoretical or intellectual virtue. However, it always involves an ability to assess relevant aspects of a situation requiring intellectual skills. While experience of a range of different situations cultivates *phronesis*, it includes being able to think beyond concrete situations.

Phronesis (and virtues in general) has an emotional component. According to Aristotle, it is a matter of learning to experience appropriate feelings of joy and pain. These feelings will contribute to good choices of action. The realisation that emotions influence action, albeit sometimes implicitly, resonates with contemporary psychological research. One example is the somatic marker hypothesis. It suggests that we learn by experience because we receive somatic feedback signalling the expected outcome of a choice of action (Ohira, 2010). This, in turn, helps us navigate complex situations. *Phronesis*, in other words, employs all means for choosing a good course of action in complex situations. At the same time, it is also partly a matter of cultivating good habits that make the more automated parts of the decision process function better.

Phronesis functions as an overarching coordinating virtue in psychotherapy. It includes the coordination of the virtues corresponding to the three components of evidence-based practice in psychology in a clinical act. Moreover, the clinical expert must possess capacities that correspond to the three components. These virtues can be described as follows:

- Best available research evidence – Epistemic virtues
- Clinical expertise – Self-reflexive virtues
- Patients' characteristics, culture, and preferences – Relational virtues

Epistemic virtues

Epistemic virtue theory integrates facts and values (Sosa, 1980). A basic premise within epistemic virtue theory is that we value truth; something important is at stake when we talk about truth and falsity (Zagzebski, 1996). As we value truth and associate certain features of a person with the ability to know what is true, we value these features. The epistemic virtues are capacities and motivation that enable us to know the truth. In psychotherapy, this is typically a matter of having knowledge that may contribute to helping the patient to achieve a better life. In other words, knowledge where facts and values are integrated.

There are two particularly prominent traditions within epistemic virtue theory. One is called 'reliabilism' and the other is called 'responsibilism.' Zagzebski (1996) has written about epistemic virtues, in general terms. Waring (2016) has addressed epistemic virtues with a view to psychotherapy more specifically. Both authors position themselves between reliabilism and responsibilism. The combination is well suited for addressing the most central epistemic challenges in psychotherapy.

'Reliabilism' defines epistemic virtues as 'cognitive tools that enable the inquirer to attain the truth more often than not' (Waring, 2016, p. 36). The cognitive tools enable the actor to pose the right questions, seek out the relevant sources of knowledge, and (on this basis) draw the right conclusions. One example is knowledge about the relationship between interventions and outcomes in psychotherapy. This does not only require 'cognitive tools' that make the actor able to understand theoretical concepts and psychotherapeutic methods. It includes insights about research methods. No single method can provide exhaustive knowledge about psychological phenomena; all methods have complementary strengths and weaknesses. In Waring's (2016) definition, the requirement for an epistemic virtue is that one should know what the case is 'more often than not.' This is a relatively unambitious goal. It is, of course, hard to establish precisely how often the actor should reach the right conclusions. This is connected to a degree of phenomenal complexity and epistemic specificity. Another issue is connected to the question of what is at stake. If we are to intervene in matters of health and well-being, we want good margins – probably well beyond 'more often than not.'

Responsibilism emphasises: '[…] the intellectual habits and dispositions to the active agency of those who seek the truth through inquiry' (Waring, 2016, p. 36). Responsibilism highlights the importance of a critical assessment of the information acquired. One example could be capacities to assess whether healthcare research is reliable. Another example could be the ability to qualify statements. The primary difference between the two traditions is in emphasis. 'Reliabilists' place greater emphasis on the outcome (i.e., the ability to know the truth). 'Responsibilists' emphasise the knowledge process (i.e., the active and critical questioning).

Psychology is a complex science which is epistemologically and methodologically diverse. The complexity of human beings makes it difficult to produce high-quality science. Therefore, it is appropriate to maintain a critical approach towards scientific findings. The two traditions 'reliabilism' and 'responsibilism' provide a balance between acquiring scientific knowledge and the critical questioning of that knowledge. This also involves a critical approach to lapses in knowledge, such as the relatively underdeveloped nosology or questionable research practices (Bohart et al., 1998; Gupta, 2014; Jackson, 2017; Melchert, 2016; Westen et al., 2004). This makes integrity and intellectual sincerity two examples of epistemic virtues. Both virtues reflect a genuine wish to understand how the world really is. In contrast, some might focus on strategic short-term benefits in promoting a given psychotherapy school or intervention.

The field of psychotherapy has been and still is riddled with relatively strong tensions between different schools of psychotherapy (Fernandez-Alvarez et al., 2016; Woolfolk, 2015). Researchers and practitioners alike often become attached to one specific psychotherapy school (Woolfolk, 2015). This comes with a risk that models are used in an inflexible way, what is known as interpretative force fitting. Interpretative force fitting entails presupposing that a model explains a phenomenon, rather than asking whether the model explains the phenomenon (Waring, 2016). This tendency makes curiosity and objectivity two important epistemic virtues in psychotherapy.

Psychotherapy contains deep levels of fact and value integration (Berg & Slaattelid, 2017). This makes understanding – here, as opposed to knowing mere facts – another therapeutic virtue. To understand means to be able to situate the knowledge and science within a greater whole, not just historically and culturally, but also practically and ethically. Understanding is crucial for good practical application of knowledge because this knowledge is to be used in a concrete situation with a concrete patient, which also requires a deeper reflection of the patient's characteristics, culture, and (most importantly) preferences.

Self-reflexive virtues

The next component of evidence-based practice in psychology is clinical expertise. The function of clinical expertise in evidence-based practice in psychology is twofold. On the one hand, the clinical expert must integrate the three components. On the other, the clinical expertise is a component to be integrated. The clinical expert must integrate knowledge about themselves with 'best available research evidence' and 'patients' characteristics, culture, and preferences.' The virtues denoting the reflection of the clinical expert are self-reflexive. Self-reflective virtues are the therapist's ability to reflect and integrate their own knowledge and experience in a good way. To describe the relevant capacities, it is necessary to take a closer look at some of the most relevant characteristics of therapists in psychotherapy. This may, however, only be determined through a brief outline of the human capacity of self-reflexivity and of psychotherapy as activity.

As humans, we probably have a unique potential for understanding ourselves and to think about our 'own subjectivity, psychic states, and traits, including one's character' (Radden & Sadler, 2010, p. 123). We are even able to be self-reflexive while acting and correct actions that do not reflect our intentions or values (Hamilton, 2013). Assessments of patients and therapeutic interventions (at least partly) reflect the therapist's values and psychological state. Some examples that affect the clinical work are personality, morality, ethical conviction, epistemic conviction, and socio-cultural background. Therefore, a hermeneutic reflection on how the therapist understands is relevant. In many contexts, a hermeneutic reflection of how the psychotherapist understands may be just as informative as what the therapist understands (Woolfolk, 2015). This may at times overlap with elements of the epistemic virtues described above.

Another strong argument for focusing on self-reflexivity is that it leads to a deeper personal integration. Personal integration illustrates why desire is included in the understanding of virtues. In psychotherapy, one may connect personal integration to therapeutic virtues as genuineness and wholeheartedness. Psychotherapy consists of a range of subtle micro processes (Stern et al., 1998). Personal integration, congruence, and wholeheartedness potentially reduce the number of blind spots in therapy and thereby reduce the likelihood of negative processes in psychotherapy (Hayes, Gelso, Goldberg, & Kivlighan, 2018; Safran & Kraus, 2014; Safran & Muran, 2000). The pan-theoretical conception of countertransference illustrates the relevance of personal integration. Hayes et al. (2018) define countertransference as 'internal and external reactions in which unresolved conflicts of the therapist, usually but not always unconscious' (p. 497). Deep self-reflexivity neutralises the risk that (typically) unconscious processes impact therapy negatively. Another important self-reflexive virtue is moderation. Many desires are incompatible with the role as psychotherapist. These are damaging to the extent that they may lead the therapist away from the fundamental aim to improve the patient's life. This makes selflessness an important therapeutic virtue (Pellegrino & Thomasma, 1993; Radden & Sadler, 2010).

Waring (2016) argues that the patient's and the therapist's virtues are intertwined. Human virtues exist in the interplay with other humans who know, care for, and challenge us. Psychotherapy often cultivates the patient's virtues. Self-reflexive virtues play an important role in treatment because internalisation of the therapist or modelling may be a part of the treatment (Aron, 1996; Goldfried, Burckell, & Eubanks-Carter, 2003). A therapist who signals that it is important to know oneself may inspire the patient to do the same. This is yet another reason why the self-reflexivity of the clinical expert holds clinical importance. We can also note that this overlaps with relational virtues to some extent.

Relational virtues

The final component, patients' characteristics, culture, and preferences, corresponds to relational virtues. Relational virtues are crucial in psychotherapeutic practice. According to virtue ethical doctrine, one should only treat identical cases alike (Aristotle, 2009). Patient's preferences vary. Thus, patients differ in ethically and clinically significant ways. Waring (2016) has argued that an integration of facts and values has a narratological function in psychotherapy Understanding how facts and values of life are interconnected is therapeutically significant if:

> It can help to organize and reconfigure what patients already know about themselves [...] [in] a "larger web of values" [where they can create] [...] a vision of what it would mean for them to live well.
>
> (Waring, 2016, p. 48)

The ability to make decisions is crucial to living well. Radden and Sadler (2010) argue that: patient autonomy has become one of the most [...] widely honoured principles within biomedical ethics (p. 114). Autonomy is often connected to duty ethics, which emphasises formalised rules for ethical conduct. At first glance, formalisation seems incompatible with the approximate nature of *phronesis*. According to Pellegrino and Thomasma (1993), it is, however, *phronesis* that makes it possible to implement duties in clinical practice. A particularly central obstacle to autonomy in psychotherapy is the power-imbalance between the therapist and the patient. Any regulatory principle must be contextualised to a specific therapeutic relation. The therapist and the patient together deal with obstacles to patient autonomy. This involves, amongst other things, an awareness of potential power-imbalances.

To create an autonomous patient, the clinical expert must be able to create a space where the patient is willing to explore their characteristics, culture, and preferences together with another person. This makes reliability a central therapeutic virtue (Pellegrino & Thomasma, 1993; Radden & Sadler, 2010). Another important relational virtue is empathy or compassion, which is the ability to grasp, and to some extent feel, what the patient feels. Since psychotherapy is emotionally demanding, perseverance and robustness are central relational virtues. Additionally, the therapist must be attentive and capable of knowing when to identify, clarify, nuance, challenge, accept, or praise any given patient. Patients may have a greater or lesser degree of awareness about their own culture, characteristics, and preferences, which is necessary for a patient to become autonomous. Therefore, perseverance and patience are relevant therapeutic virtues (Radden & Sadler, 2010).

Therapeutic virtues

Because psychotherapy is a complex practice, a vast number of therapeutic virtues are relevant. It would be far beyond the scope of this chapter to provide a complete list of all relevant virtues. The main point is not exclusively that virtue ethics is relevant for psychotherapy. Importantly, it can help us to clarify how the different components in evidence-based practice in psychology may result in good practice. The other main point is that virtue ethics indicates that the clinical integration starts with the particular (i.e., the individual patient) and is informed by the three components of evidence-based practice in psychology. It also makes the therapist accountable.

A common objection towards virtue ethics is that it is perfectionistic. In this context, this means that one poses unrealistic expectations towards what characterises competent therapists. It is, however, important to distinguish between ideals and realistic expectations of professionals. Establishing a regulatory principle that functions as an ideal can entail an acceptance that one may fail to reach these ideals. Of course, it is hard to define perfection in a practice like psychotherapy. The patients' needs and goals are individual. On the one hand, this may be a source of frustration. On the other, it may be a remedy for rigid ideals. Psychotherapy based on *phronesis* seeks to distance itself from sterile thinking. Good treatment, which includes the relevant parameters, is particular and individual. This does not, however, mean that 'anything goes.' Quite the opposite: it means that one must be more precise and thorough than one would need to be if one relied exclusively on scientific evidence.

The ultimate aim of psychotherapy is to create a better life for patients. The patient is at the centre of what good psychotherapy means. The ideal is not paternalistic. The integrating psychotherapists base themselves on the patient's preferences and inform the patient to become autonomous. It is also important to emphasise that psychotherapy is a relational activity which functions as an active collaboration. A conceptualisation of psychotherapy based on *phronesis* is highly compatible with a such a notion of psychotherapy. This makes it possible to approach the patient's own goals. Regardless of whether the problem is clear to the patient initially or time is needed to establish an understanding of the problem.

Conclusion

If evidence-based practice in psychology is to be an integration conducted by a clinical expert, the clinical expert must possess some capacities to integrate. These are the therapeutic virtues. A focus on therapeutic virtues will have implications for the education of psychotherapists. We have seen in Chapter 3 that one of the most important rationales for evidence-based medicine was the training of medical students. A model based on virtue ethics will focus on the therapist's capacities that contribute to helping the patients they meet as individuals. This does not only entail an understanding of research literature and of the meanings and limitations of research literature. It also includes the ability to identify the individual patient's unique values. This, furthermore, entails an awareness of the impact the therapist themself has on the psychotherapy and an ability to integrate this in therapeutic considerations and actions. In many ways, this is a far more demanding ideal that to learn to read research literature, but it is also an ideal which to corresponds to the conceptual and the empirical knowledge on psychotherapy. The distinctive character of the practice must decide the parameters for best practice. The revised virtue-based model is founded on psychotherapy itself and to a lesser extent based on strategic thinking. Therefore, this regulatory principle will also be a lot more expedient with regard to the fundamental goal of psychotherapy: to create a better life for the patient in treatment.

References

Aristotle. 2009. The Nicomachean Ethics. Translated by David Ross and Lesley Brown, *Oxford World's Classics*. Oxford: Oxford University Press.

Aron, L. (1996). *A meeting of minds: Mutuality in psychoanalysis*. Mahwah, NJ: The Analytic Press.

Berg, H. (2020). Virtue ethics and integration in evidence-based practice in psychology. *Frontiers in Psychology, 11*(258). http://doi.org/10.3389/fpsyg.2020.00258

Berg, H., & Slaattelid, R. 2017. Facts and values in psychotherapy: A critique of the empirical reduction of psychotherapy within evidence-based practice. *Journal of Evaluation in Clinical Practice 23*(5), 1075–1080. http://doi.org/10.1111/jep.12739

Bohart, Arthur C., O'Hara, Maureen, & Leitner, Larry M.. 1998. Empirically violated treatments: Disenfranchisement of humanistic and other psychotherapies. *Psychotherapy Research 8*(2), 141–157. http://doi.org/10.1080/10503309812331332277

Cochrane, A.L. 1999. *Effectiveness and efficiency: Random reflections on health services*. London: Royal Society of Medicine Press.

Fernandez-Alvarez, H., Consoli, A. J., & Gomez, B.. 2016. Integration in psychotherapy: Reasons and challenges. *American Psychologist 71*(8), 820–830. http://doi.org/10.1037/amp0000100

Goldfried, M. R., Burckell, L. A., & Eubanks-Carter, C. (2003). Therapist self-disclosure in cognitive-behavior therapy. *Journal of Clinical Psychology*, *59*(5), 555–568. http://doi.org/10.1002/jclp.10159

Gupta, M. (2014). *Is evidence-based psychiatry ethical?* Oxford: Oxford University Press.

Hamilton, R. (2013). The frustrations of virtue: The myth of moral neutrality in psychotherapy. *Journal of Evaluation in Clinical Practice*, *19*(3), 485–492. http://doi.org/10.1111/jep.12044

Hayes, J. A., Gelso, C. J., Goldberg, S., & Kivlighan, D. M. (2018). Countertransference management and effective psychotherapy: Meta-analytic findings. *Psychotherapy*, *55*(4), 496–507. http://doi.org/10.1037/pst0000189

Hengartner, M. P. (2018). Raising awareness for the replication crisis in clinical psychology by focusing on inconsistencies in psychotherapy research: How much can we rely on published findings from efficacy trials? *Frontiers in Psychology*. http://doi.org/10.3389/fpsyg.2018.00256

Jackson, M. R. 2017. Unified clinical science, or paradigm diversity?: Comment on Melchert. *American psychologist 72*(4), 395–396. doi: http://doi.org/10.1037/amp0000125

Levant, Ronald F. 2005. Report of the 2005 Presidential Task Force on evidence-based practice. edited by American Psychological Association.

Melchert, T. P. 2016. Leaving behind our preparadigmatic past: Professional psychology as a unified clinical science. *American Psychologist 71*(6), 486–496. http://doi.org/10.1037/a004022

Norcross, John C., Hogan, Thomas P., and Koocher, Gerald P.. 2008. *Clinician's guide to evidence based practices: Mental health and the addictions, Clinician"s Guide to Evidence Based Practices*. New York, NY: Oxford University Press.

Ohira, H. (2010). The somatic marker revisited: Brain and body in emotional decision making. *Emotion Review*, *2*(3), 245–249. http://doi.org/10.1177/1754073910362599

Pellegrino, Edmund D., & Thomasma, David C. 1993. *The virtues in medical practice*. New York, NY: Oxford University Press.

Radden, J., & Sadler, J. Z. (2010). *The virtuous psychiatrist: Character ethics in psychiatric practice*. Oxford: Oxford University Press.

Safran, J. D., & Kraus, J. (2014). Alliance ruptures, impasses, and enactments: A relational perspective. *Psychotherapy*, *51*(3), 381–387. http://doi.org/10.1037/a0036815

Safran, J. D., & Muran, J. C. (2000). *Negotiating the therapeutic alliance*. New York, NY: The Guilford Press.

Sosa, E. (1980). The Raft and the Pyramid: Coherence versus Foundations in the Theory of Knowledge. *Midwest Studies in Philosophy*, *5*(1), 3–26.

Stern, D. N., Bruschweiler-Stern, N., Harrison, A. M., Lyons-Ruth, K., Morgan, A. C., Nahum, J. P., … Tronick, E. Z. (1998). The process of therapeutic change involving implicit knowledge: Some implications of developmental observations for adult psychotherapy. *Infant Mental Health Journal*, *19*(3), 300–308.

Timmermans, Stefan, & Berg, Marc. 2003. *The gold standard: The challenge of evidence-based medicine and standardization in health care*. Philadelphia, PA: Temple University Press.

Waring, Duff R. 2016. *The healing virtues*. Oxford: Oxford University Press.

Waterman, A. S. (2008). Reconsidering happiness: A eudaimonist's perspective. *The Journal of Positive Psychology*, *3*(4), 234–252. http://doi.org/10.1080/17439760802303002

Westen, D., Novotny, C. M., & Thompson-Brenner, H. 2004. The empirical status of empirically supported psychotherapies: Assumptions, findings, and reporting in controlled clinical trials. *The Psychological Bulletin 130*(4), 631–63. http://doi.org/10.1037/0033-2909.130.4.631

Woolfolk, Robert L. 2015. *The value of psychotherapy: The talking cure in an age of clinical science*. New York, NY: The Guilford Press.

Zagzebski, L. T. (1996). *Virtues of the mind: An inquiry into the nature of virtue and the ethical foundations of knowledge*. Cambridge: Cambridge University Press.

Zarkovich, E., & Upshur, R. E. G. (2002). The virtues of evidence. *Theoretical Medicine*, *23*, 403–412. http://doi.org/10.1023/A:1021217908383

9 Conclusion

This book has addressed the central tenets and the developmental history of evidence-based practice in psychology. Evidence-based practice in psychology rests upon problematic presuppositions. Many of the philosophical traditions that have informed evidence-based practice in psychology have either been discarded or are highly contested. The same holds true for the political ideals. There is reason to believe that other considerations than quality of treatment have played a part in keeping these ideals alive.

The developmental history clearly shows that evidence-based practice in psychology was a strategic manoeuvre. The profession wanted to ensure that psychotherapy (qua 'talking cure') would remain an alternative for people with mental illnesses. However, whereas evidence-based medicine has been revised continuously to accommodate criticism, evidence-based practice in psychology is yet to be revised. An assessment that evaluates whether the current policy statement is suited for regulating psychotherapy practice in an appropriate way is overdue.

One of the greatest problems of evidence-based practice in psychology is the conceptualisation of psychotherapy. Evidence-based practice in psychology fails to capture the distinctive character of psychotherapy. It is defined as a technical solution to a fixed problem that may be answered through science alone. Psychotherapy is, however, an ethical pursuit. The answer to the question cannot be found in criteria for diagnoses nor in research results. To be able to assess whether a given development is a good development for a given patient, we must deploy ethics.

Moreover, evidence-based practice in psychology is implicitly utilitarian. A practice is legitimate if it realises a given delimited outcome. However, psychotherapy practice is highly complex. Hence, we should have a range of ethical perspectives at our disposal to be able to illuminate different aspects of clinical practice. Ethical pluralism is the best safety net against severely unethical practices which unfortunately abound in the history of psychiatry and psychology.

Evidence-based practice should be reformulated to ensure that the principle is in accordance with the original intentions. It must become the

DOI: 10.4324/9781003512141-9

threefold model that evidence-based practice in psychology was intended to be. In this reconstruction, one must separate between 'clinical expertise' and 'patient characteristics, culture, and preferences' as objects of inquiry, and the individual clinical expertise of a psychotherapist and the individual preferences of an actual patient. This is a pressing ethical issue, not only to provide treatment adapted to each specific situation, but also to safeguard the patient's right to participation in decision-making in a good way.

Finally, it is important to connect the clinical integration to the clinical expert. At the same time, it is crucial that the clinical expert is not allowed to work unrestrictedly. The two other components (best available research evidence and patient's preferences) must have a corrective effect on the clinical expert. This will contribute to food clinical decisions and treatment for patients in need of psychotherapy. Furthermore, this will contribute to a more accountable conceptualisation of psychotherapy as a practice with a purpose of realising good individual outcomes.

Index

For Product Safety Concerns and Information please contact our EU representative GPSR@taylorandfrancis.com Taylor & Francis Verlag GmbH, Kaufingerstraße 24, 80331 München, Germany

Batch number: 10398441

Printed by Printforce, the Netherlands